Praise for Make the School System Work for Your Child with Disabilities

"Warm and accessible, this book equips you with knowledge and strategies to work with the school system to best support your child. From understanding evaluation options, to getting the most out of IEPs and 504 Plans, to collaborating with teachers and related service providers, and so much more, this book is an essential tool to help you set your child up for school success."
                    —**Lindsey Biel, MA, OTR/L, occupational**
                        therapist; coauthor of *Raising a Sensory*
                        Smart Child

"This book is a trail guide for parents navigating unfamiliar and daunting terrain. Stacey Shubitz speaks 'parent to parent' with the insights of a well-informed traveler. She guides you to become an advocate for your child, offering sage advice and extensive resources. If I could recommend only one book to help parents understand and navigate how to get support for a child with a disability, it would be this one."
                    —**Lester L. Laminack, EdD, author, consultant,**
                        and Professor Emeritus, Western Carolina
                        University

"I wish I could gift this book to every parent who has just received a diagnosis for their child or is exploring getting their child evaluated. This book is bringing back memories for me as a parent—and I am also making brand-new discoveries. Stacey Shubitz digs deeply into her own and others' experiences and shares hard-won lessons with all of us."
                    —**Samara D., Portland, Maine**

"Parents and educators reading this book will find a fierce ally, perhaps even a life coach, certainly a joy guru!"
                    —**Katherine Bomer, MA, educator, author,**
                        and consultant, Sherman, Connecticut

"A treasure chest for parents of children with disabilities and caregivers. Stacey Shubitz has packed this book with the critical information families need, as well as guidance for our entire journey. She writes with warmth, empathy, and grace, in part because she has walked this path, too. As a longtime educator and a parent of two children with IEPs, I only wish this book had been around when I first embarked on this journey, but am beyond grateful that it is here now."
                    —**M. Colleen Cruz, MA, educator, author, and**
                        consultant, New York City

MAKE THE
SCHOOL SYSTEM
WORK
FOR YOUR CHILD
WITH DISABILITIES

MAKE THE SCHOOL SYSTEM
—— WORK ——
FOR YOUR CHILD
WITH DISABILITIES

Empowering Kids for the Future

Stacey Shubitz, MSEd, MA

gp

THE GUILFORD PRESS
New York   London

Printed in the United States of America

For product and safety concerns within the EU, please contact *GPSR@taylorandfrancis.com,*
Taylor & Francis Verlag GmbH, Kaufingerstraße 24, 80331 München, Germany.

Last digit is print number: 9   8   7   6   5   4   3   2   1

This publication is intended to provide helpful and informative material. It is not intended to
diagnose, treat, cure, or prevent any health problem or condition, nor is it intended to replace the
advice of a health professional. No action should be taken based solely on the contents of this
book. Always consult your physician or qualified health care professional on any matters regarding
your health and before adopting any suggestions in this book or drawing inferences from it.

The author and publisher specifically disclaim all responsibility for any liability, loss, or risk,
personal or otherwise, which is incurred as a consequence, directly or indirectly, from the use or
application of any contents of this book.

Any and all product names referenced within this book are the trademarks of their respective
owners. Always read all information provided by the manufacturers' product labels before using
their products. The author and publisher are not responsible for claims made by manufacturers.

Library of Congress Cataloging-in-Publication Data is available from the publisher.

ISBN 978-1-4625-5413-3 (paperback) — ISBN 978-1-4625-5937-4 (hardcover)

To my dear children, you are my greatest joy.

Contents

Part Three
Embracing Opportunities: Making the Most of Nonschool Hours

Author's Note

Throughout this book, I use the term *parent* to refer collectively to all individuals who share the responsibility of caring for and raising a child. I understand families come in diverse forms and that not every child resides with their biological parents. My intention is to make this book inclusive for all families, acknowledging and respecting the unique family structure of each reader.

I have put in my best effort to include the most up-to-date information to help you navigate the special education system at your child's public school. I consulted people with more knowledge than I have in specific areas. I attempted to craft a book to help most parents, but I will be the first to admit that I am an imperfect human. And, although any parent can find value in the book's content, please note that certain aspects may not be relevant if your child is enrolled in a private or parochial school or is receiving their education outside the United States.

Given the changes proposed to the U.S. Department of Education in 2025, it's important to remember that special education laws and mandates evolve and change. Therefore, there will be new things to discover about this topic soon after its publication. You may have to do additional research to help answer specific questions about the special education rules in your state. The world of disability itself is also ever-evolving, and while I strive to use proper terminology and explanations throughout this book, some information may have changed since this book's publication date.

While I respect my child's privacy and do not discuss her medical information with strangers, she has permitted me to share some things about her life. However, I am mindful to share in a way that maintains a strong and respectful relationship with my daughter. I assure you that I uphold the same level of respect for all children and individuals mentioned in this book.

Preserving confidentiality is paramount. The stories I present in this book are all accurate. In many cases, I have created composite characters, and in others, I have altered names and other identifying characteristics to protect the privacy of children and other individuals described.

I've strived to use language that reflects current inclusive practices. Sometimes you'll notice terms that are outdated or not aligned with current best practices in inclusive language; these examples reflect terms still used in some educational settings. My use of these terms is not an endorsement of such language but a reflection of existing institutional norms.

Acknowledgments

Thank you, reader, for investing your time and energy in this book as you seek to support your child more effectively. Your commitment to their well-being is commendable. I appreciate you joining me to celebrate the incredible people who helped make this book happen.

To the wonderful people at The Guilford Press, I am grateful you believed in this book and made it a reality. Kitty Moore saw the potential in this project upon reading my book proposal. Jason Matloff and Kitty met with me on Zoom to discuss the possibilities of this book proposal. I knew I had found the right home for my book since we discussed writing and New York baseball from day one. My developmental editor, Christine Benton, gave me thoughtful and honest feedback. I have always valued Chris's perspective and the encouragement she has offered to help me improve my writing. After I was diagnosed with breast cancer in late 2024, Chris did everything she could to guide the manuscript from my computer to the copyeditor, ensuring that no time was wasted. Thank you for understanding and respecting my needs as a person and a writer during those months. You have my heartfelt gratitude. I am appreciative of Melissa Raymond for the care she put into producing this book. I am grateful for both your kindness and your incredible troubleshooting skills! I am deeply grateful to Samantha Grossman for her meticulous and dedicated work overseeing the permissions process. Many thanks to Anna Brackett and Judith Grauman for their keen eyes and attention to detail. I am grateful to Monica Baum for shaping the marketing campaign with creativity and insight and to Lucy Baker for guiding the book's publicity with care and creativity.

To my generous colleagues, who helped me bring this book to life and onto the page. Bill Varner, who edited my books for Stenhouse Publishers, listened as I shared my initial concept and helped me realize that I had a book intended for families, not teachers, forming in my mind. He made himself available to answer my questions even though we no longer worked as editor and writer. Leah Mermelstein posed questions that guided me in further refining my idea by reviewing an early draft of the book proposal and offering me valuable insights on later chapters. Lynne Dorfman encouraged me as I dipped into writing for an audience beyond classroom teachers and literacy coaches. Everyone deserves the steadfast support of colleagues like Lynne, who has become, as my son puts it, "part of our family." Melanie Meehan, with whom I co-host the Two Writing Teachers Podcast, has been an invaluable thought partner for over a decade. She kindly reviewed several chapters and discussed various issues with me as the deadline for submitting the manuscript approached.

It was an honor to teach upper elementary students, and I'm grateful for them. During my years in the classroom, I learned a tremendous amount about life, advocacy, and care. Teaching has taught me that wisdom flows in all directions—from teacher to student and in a complex, beautiful reciprocity.

My colleagues from Two Writing Teachers have helped me grow as an educator, thinker, and writer. Two Writing Teachers has been a labor of love since its inception, and I'm grateful I have gotten to write and think alongside members of the coauthor team, past and present. In addition, I am thankful to the Slice of Life community, which meets on Tuesdays year-round and daily in March on Two Writing Teachers. You have helped me grow as a writer, educator, and parent. You've cheered me on and have pushed my thinking. I am grateful to all of you for reading my words and commenting with care.

I am deeply grateful to the remarkable speech, occupational, physical, and music therapists who have been instrumental in my development as a parent. I want to express my gratitude to Lynn Cummings, Jill Henig, Joanna Kirby, Megan Klinger-Satterwhite, Marie Kurtz, Karen Reale, Mandy Rudy, and Jena Shovlin for your unwavering support, commitment, and expertise during my early years as a parent. Your dedication made a profound difference. You have had a positive impact on many children's lives. Thank you for all you do!

I'm endlessly grateful to Dr. Jill M. Eckert, Dr. Paul M. Haidet, Dr. Kristine L. Widders, Dr. Timothy S. Johnson, Dr. Raymond J. Hohl, Hope Yusko, and Soyoung Baek, who ensured my health and stamina while working on this book. Your care made it possible for me to bring this project to life.

I thank Cynthia Adams, Diana Autin, Lori Butterfield, Robyn Chotiner, Samara Cole Doyon, Carrie Ferguson, Amy Fisher, Deb Frazier, Lydia Glore, Betsy Hubbard, Kabrillen Jones, Susan Kennedy, Abi Luger, Danielle McGhee, Kendall McKinney, Amber Mentz, Arlynn Paris, Heatherann Paul,

Jen Patenaude, Beth Rementer, Melanie Ribich, Marina Rodriguez, Debbie Sasson, Maureen Stabler, Dan Stewart, Jeff Sullivan, Lyon Terry, and Kyle Vercammen for answering my questions and generously sharing your expertise with me.

I appreciate several strong women I've grown with and leaned on for many years. I treasure each of you: Alexa Andewelt, Stacey Nolish Blank, Jackie Hafter, Rachel Mandelman, Marcela Moschcovich, and Emily Kretchmer Winthrop. You are the source of laughter, comfort, and strength. Thank you for being there to celebrate the good times and to lift me in darker hours.

I thank my cousin William Kevorkian, for encouraging me to find the right home for this book. I will always be grateful for your frankness and your wisdom! Jared Peet and Annie Infantino, I appreciate your perspective and knowledge as educators. Just as your students are lucky to have you as their teachers, I am fortunate to have you as my cousins!

My fruzzins, Scott Shubitz and Tiffany Hensley, have always been willing to listen, read, and provide feedback to me. I am grateful for your unwavering support and the way you can always make me laugh, even on the bleakest days. I wish we lived closer, but cherish all the pebbling we do to stay close.

My parents, Marcia and Gerald Shubitz, deserve a ticker-tape parade in their honor for their dedication to me, my husband, and our children. While writing this book, my family of four endured six surgeries. My parents dropped everything *four times* in less than two years to come help us out, sometimes for months at a time. Thank you for being a source of stability when it felt like everything was out of control. While I'm thankful for the time we've spent together, I sincerely hope you'll enjoy your retirement even more in the years to come. I love you both.

To my children: I remember having lunch with you a few months ago at one of our favorite restaurants. We talked about the places we had visited and the trips we hoped to take. That lunch stands out in my mind even now—it was a time without any arguments, filled with your happiness over your meal, and the excitement you felt about traveling together as a family. Like all siblings, you two often disagree, but that conversation has lingered with me. It is a beautiful reminder of your love for each other and our family. I know this past year has posed many challenges, especially as the words *the book* and *cancer* became frequent parts of our conversations. I love you both and want you to know how grateful I am to have you as my children. My heart feels full when we're all together, and now that we've come through the other side of it, I'm excited for more outings and adventures. Let's explore and see what amazing things we can find!

Marc Schaefer is the greatest supporter of my writing life. He understands he shouldn't interrupt me if I'm wearing my reading glasses and typing furiously, since that means I'm in the writing zone. He ferries the kids out of the house to give me quiet time on Sundays when he knows it's been a busy week. He reminds me when it's getting late and helps me close down the computer at night so I get the rest I need. I am grateful for your love and friendship. I could not ask for more.

Introduction
Get Oriented

My heart raced with hope and trepidation when I walked my daughter into school for her first day of kindergarten. With her hand in mine, we navigated the hallways, the hubbub, and the terrain of a world not entirely built for her unique needs. As we approached her classroom, her teacher greeted us. After finding her cubby and seeing familiar faces, my daughter shooed me off. While I was relieved not to deal with tears, I felt a surge of conflicting emotions—relief, anxiety, and determination—for what was to come: a journey that would expand my understanding of parenthood, education, advocacy, and the myriad ways we all learn and grow.

My child's educational journey has been defined not by perfection but by persistent curiosity and adaptability. Throughout this experience, I've learned that setbacks are not endpoints but opportunities for reimagining what's possible. The strong foundation built during her elementary school years has enabled her to thrive as much as any middle schooler can during one of life's most challenging stages. However, it's important to acknowledge that our path has had its fair share of obstacles.

In this book, I share my experiences as an educator and parent of a school-age child, hoping to support those in a similar situation to the one I found myself in when my child entered elementary school. My journey has been continuous learning—listening, observing, researching, and asking questions. This book won't have all the answers, nor will it be a "one size fits all" approach. I aim to provide insights and strategies that have been valuable to me as I've navigated the educational landscape as a parent.

I write with a deep understanding of the complex emotions that often accompany our children's educational journeys. I've learned that challenges can be addressed through advocacy, collaboration, and persistence. There are always possibilities for positive change. Parents can take plenty of action to ensure their children receive the education they need and deserve so they can excel in their journey through school.

HOW IT STARTED

I met my husband, Marc, when I was living in Manhattan in my late twenties. After a brief stint in Rhode Island, we settled in Pennsylvania. Our daughter was born three years after we married. She was an adorable, albeit colicky, baby. I loved every ounce of her. I knew early on that she wasn't reaching developmental milestones like the other kids in the Mommy & Me Group I attended for the first year of her life.

Despite having a loving family and excellent physicians and therapists who worked with our daughter, I felt alone as I navigated my daughter's early years. Some friends were supportive, but many didn't understand my daily struggles. I distanced myself from friends who didn't try to understand my daughter when she spoke. I retreated from anyone who said, "Einstein was three when he started speaking."

I started a support group at a nearby hospital for parents whose children had the same motor-speech disorder. It comforted me to talk with other parents whose kids were struggling like mine, but it wasn't enough since the group met bimonthly. I still felt lost, lonely, and exhausted.

HOW IT'S GOING

I turned this book in to my publisher while my daughter was in eighth grade. She has accommodations written into her Individualized Education Program (IEP), but she spends 100% of her school day in a general education setting. We still deal with complex issues, but I'm better equipped to handle them now that I've walked through her early and middle childhood years. Despite watching my daughter thrive as she entered middle school, I do not have everything sorted out. I am a human being who is continuously expanding my understanding and who doesn't have all the answers. I've acquired tools along the way, and they've helped me continue to navigate our lives every time I feel like we've been dinged or knocked down.

I have been involved in and driven to countless appointments, neuropsych evaluations, tutoring sessions, IEP meetings, and medical visits. As a parent,

I have navigated private and public schools. It has been challenging, but I've found ways to keep life joyful as we've muddled through the messiness.

I'm an educator by profession. I'm a certified literacy specialist and a former fourth- and fifth-grade teacher who has worked as a literacy consultant focusing on writing workshop in grades K–6. I've published three books for teachers and a writing workshop curriculum for grades 2–5. In addition, I am a blogger and a podcaster who focuses on—wait for it—the teaching of writing. On the personal front, I'm a wife and mother to two children who are about six years apart. Whenever I have downtime, I enjoy activities such as baking, reading, swimming, practicing Pilates, and taking long walks.

WHAT'S INSIDE THIS BOOK

I hope this book will be a steadfast companion, offering you a roadmap to navigate your child's elementary school years. The book is organized into three parts, where you'll learn about the special education landscape, how to prepare for an IEP meeting, how to advocate for accommodations, and more.

An overview of what's ahead:

- Part I: Advocacy in Action: Transforming Obstacles into Opportunities—*You'll begin by considering your child's needs. I'll help you learn how to meet them by getting concrete answers about your child's disability.*

  o Chapter 1: Identify Needs and Lead with Strengths—Accept and embrace your child's disability as an essential part of their identity. Learn about various disability types and adopt a strengths-based approach highlighting your child's capabilities rather than limitations.

  o Chapter 2: Chart Your Course through the Evaluation Process—Trust your instincts and advocate for a comprehensive educational evaluation. Familiarize yourself with the school evaluation process and understand how to foster collaborative partnerships.

- Part II: Navigating the Education Maze: Maximizing Your Child's Education—*In the heart of this book, I'll help you maneuver through the intricacies of your child's schooling.*

  o Chapter 3: Become Familiar with the Landscape—Navigate the special education landscape by understanding the differences between IEPs and 504 Plans—and how each supports students' needs—and discovering the various service providers who support students with disabilities.

o Chapter 4: Know What Your Child Will Receive—Explore critical special education services and advocate for your child's unique learning needs by understanding the Least Restrictive Environment (LRE) principle and how it impacts educational support.

o Chapter 5: Strengthen Learning through Customized Instruction—Delve into Specially Designed Instruction (SDI) and understand how educators can tailor learning experiences for students with disabilities using a variety of supports, accommodations, and modifications.

o Chapter 6: Prepare, Partner, and Advocate for IEP Meeting Success—Prepare for your child's IEP meeting with confidence by gathering information, creating personalized documents, and establishing rapport with educators to advocate effectively for your child's needs.

o Chapter 7: Communicate with Teachers and School Staff—Learn how to initiate effective communication with your child's teachers and staff to foster a collaborative partnership and address your child's unique educational needs.

• Part III: Embracing Opportunities: Making the Most of Nonschool Hours—*I'll help you find ways to enrich your home life, empowering yourself and your child.*

o Chapter 8: Curate Joy—Discover practical tips and personal insights for bringing more joy into your and your child's life. This chapter offers strategies for navigating various situations and fostering positive experiences in your family's journey.

o Chapter 9: The Power of Reading Together—Explore the benefits of sharing books as a family, from fostering language development to strengthening bonds. Discover recommended inclusive literature, including books that feature representation of various disabilities, to promote compassion, understanding, and a sense of belonging.

o Chapter 10: Teach Self-Advocacy—Empower your child to advocate for their needs by exploring common challenges and providing strategies that foster their self-advocacy skills in various contexts.

o Afterword: Take Care of Yourself—This note to you provides guidance on prioritizing self-care throughout your parenting journey.

It delves into authentic self-care for parents juggling various obligations, emphasizing that nurturing your well-being will leave you well-rested and ready to advocate for your child.

At the end of the book, you'll find relevant resources to help you go deeper into the topics covered in each chapter. Plus, resources are available at *www.guilford.com/shubitz-materials* that you may duplicate for personal use.

Additional Features You'll Find in Every Chapter

- **Tips:** On the day a renowned speech-language pathologist confirmed my daughter's childhood apraxia of speech diagnosis, he provided various suggestions to help her speak better. He also gave us sage advice: "Take care of your marriage." I looked at him with bewilderment. How would that help our daughter put words together to make intelligible sentences? He explained that we would be drained from pouring ourselves into helping her. He emphasized the importance of self-care and making time to be a couple, not just as co-parents. It turned out to be some of the best advice we've received since we learned the importance of nurturing our relationship.

  This is a parenting book, not a self-help book. *But* I know you must take care of yourself, which is why each chapter contains a self-care tip and a tip for cultivating joy. I've walked this road and know that you cannot care for your child well if you aren't actively caring for yourself and making time to enjoy the life you have.

- **Vignettes:** I will illustrate points throughout the book by sharing stories from my journey, as well as the stories of others. All of the people involved have been disguised to protect their privacy.

  If you connect to something you read, you might jot down your own story in a journal or on a document on your computer. Writing is cathartic. Plus, you never know how a vignette you write today could help a friend or family member in the future when they're experiencing something similar.

  This book holds significance as a resource not only for you but also for me. I anticipate returning to it repeatedly whenever I need it. I hope you, too, will use it as a toolbox that offers strategies and solutions—plus support—needed for specific issues that arise throughout your journey.

HOW TO USE THIS BOOK

Please begin with chapter one before moving on to the rest of the book . . . even if you have an IEP meeting tomorrow! After that, choose a chapter that fits with the challenges you're facing right now. Then spend time implementing what you're learning and applying it to empower yourself as a parent. You may read this book cover to cover, then return to parts of it based on what you need in the future.

Break out a writing utensil and some sticky notes or a device. Make notes on the pages and tab anything you want to return to. You might want to schedule an email to yourself with something you want to remember in the future, or record a voice memo on your phone. Hold on to the information you glean from these pages in whatever way will be helpful to you and your child.

As I've said, getting support for your child with disabilities to thrive in school can feel very isolating. It's also confusing because, while federal legal protections are currently in place, states and communities within them vary in what they offer. See the box on pages 6–8 for important resources you can start accessing right now.

Variations in the Disability World
Finding State and Local Help

Every state does different things to help students with disabilities. It's impossible to write a book that covers all the existing nuances. However, there are some constants.

Legal protections stem from the Individuals with Disabilities Education Act (IDEA). The IDEA protects any student who receives special education. You'll often hear these legal protections referred to as *procedural safeguards*. School districts provide parents with a list of procedural safeguards, which help inform you of your rights and what you can expect as you go through the evaluation and IEP process. Typically, schools will provide this to you in writing, but you can ask for a verbal explanation of the safeguards if you need clarification.

There is a network of Parent Centers across the country. Every state has a **Parent Training and Information Center, or PTI**, to improve the educational outcomes of people up to 26 years of age with disabilities. The PTIs provide free courses, training, links to support groups, and information to families. There are also 26 **Community Parent Resource Centers (CPRCs)** nationwide. Every state has at least one Parent Center, as found on the Center for Parent Information and Resources (CPIR) website. CPIR maintains state-by-state listings of PTIs and CPRCs. (Find a PTI or CPRC near you: *www.parentcenterhub.org/find-your-center.*) Parent Centers provide families with free information and resources to help them build their capacity to advocate for their child with disabilities. They hold webinars, share resources, provide programming in special education topics, and provide trainings. They also maintain active lists of free or low-cost attorneys and advocates.

Family-to-Family Health Information Centers (F2Fs) are organizations led by families, providing assistance and guidance to families of children with disabilities and special health care needs. F2Fs can help you navigate the health system or help you work with your school district if your child's health-related issues impact their education. There are 59 F2Fs, with at least one in every state. (Find your local F2F by scrolling down and clicking on the map: *https://familyvoices.org.*)

The National Federation of Families has a network of affiliates that support families with a child who has mental health issues or substance use. This organization provides peer support and support services. It also provides information on your rights for your children's care, tips for getting referrals, trainings, and many other resources. (Find your affiliate: *www.ffcmh.org/our-affiliates.*)

Parent to Parent USA is a national nonprofit organization that provides emotional support to families of individuals with disabilities or special health care needs. It operates through a network connecting parents with trained volunteers with similar experiences. Parent to Parent USA assists families by fostering connections and offering emotional support. It matches parents who need emotional support with trained mentors who provide guidance, information, resilience, and understanding. (Find a local Parent to Parent near you: *www.p2pusa.org/parents.*)

National Disability Rights Network is the membership organization for the 57 **Protection and Advocacy, or P&A**, agencies across the 50 states, all U.S. territories, and one serving the Native American population in the Four Corners. P&As help parents with advocacy, inform policymakers, and do outreach to different interest groups. They also "monitor and investigate" abuse, neglect, exploitation, or incidents that may have harmed someone with a disability. (Find the P&A in Your State: *www.ndrn.org.*)

Finally, most state education departments will have an office that provides parents with specific information about resolving disputes, answers questions about federal and state laws, and provides resources to help your child access a free and appropriate public education. A quick internet search with something like "special education consult line {state's name}" can help you find the right state-level office.

BEFORE GETTING STARTED

Plenty of books, blogs, podcasts, and websites will help you better understand your child's disability. This book will not dive deep into specific disabilities. Rather, this book is me sharing what I've learned from experts, countless hours of reading, knowledge of other parents' and educators' experiences, and my lived experiences as a classroom teacher, literacy consultant, and parent.

I may not be beside you, but I'm cheering you on from afar. Throughout the book, I introduce you to information I wish someone had shared with me at various points during my daughter's elementary school years. Let's begin with this:

Disability Is Not a Four-Letter Word

Tiffany Yu, founder of Diversability and author of *The Anti-Ableist Manifesto: Smashing Stereotypes, Forging Change, and Building a Disability-Inclusive World,* defines disability has "a health condition of the body and or mind that impacts the way a person participates in daily activities" (2024, 4). You'll notice there is not a negative value judgment by talking about disability as an impairment in Yu's definition. This is because Yu, and many within the disability community, emphasize that disability is simply one part of human diversity; it isn't something to be pitied or feared. By avoiding terms like "impairment" or "deficit," Yu's definition highlights that disability is a natural variation in the way people experience the world, not something inherently negative. This perspective shifts the conversation toward acceptance, empowerment, and inclusion.

As my daughter got older, I realized that my reluctance to discuss her disabilities openly stemmed not only from a need for privacy but also from ableism. I had internalized society's view that being disabled was a deficit, something to be cured. Perhaps this is because I came of age when society told us disability was a deficit, an issue that needed fixing. Years ago, words like *disability* and *disabled* were considered derogatory. To this day, much of society believes disability is like a "four-letter word."

But it isn't.

The disabled community has reclaimed those words, embracing disability as part of their identity. Disability Pride Month, observed in July, honors the community's rich history, accomplishments, and resilience.

Acknowledging my missteps, I embarked on a journey of education and advocacy. I delved into *own voices books* by disabled authors and followed disabled content creators on social media. In doing so, I learned from the disabled community, which is actively working to promote awareness and understanding.

We discuss disability at the dinner table, acknowledging it is part of our family life and many other people's lives. It's important to me that my children understand that people with disabilities aren't a monolith. They need to know that every person with a disability is as unique and different from each other as anyone else. We do not treat the d-word as a four-letter word. In essence, we became a disability-positive family.

YOU. ARE. POWERFUL.

Remember those superlatives (Most Congenial, Best Eyes, Cutest, etc.) you voted on at the end of middle and high school? I was voted "most responsible" at the end of eighth grade, which has always felt cringy. I recognize that I deviate from the norm. Being what some people would call "Type A" is just how I'm wired. *You* don't need to be inherently detail-oriented and organized to advocate for your child! I'll give you lists, strategies, tools, and tips to empower you to become efficient, proactive, and results-focused.

You hold power as your child's caregiver. You are their first teacher. If you've sold yourself short and thought you didn't know enough to help your child, that's about to change. You—not their teacher, principal, or doctor— know your child the best. Let's harness that power and begin!

> **Tip for Cultivating Joy:** Spending time with someone who makes you feel good gives you energy rather than depleting you. As adults, we may have friends who live far away, so remember you can connect via phone or video chat.

Self-Care Tip: Commit to practicing self-compassion so you speak to yourself in a supportive and kind way. You can nurture your soul by talking to yourself in the same way you would to someone you love unconditionally.

Part I

Advocacy in Action

Transforming Obstacles into Opportunities

1

Identify Needs and Lead with Strengths

I met Becca at a playground when our children were three and four years old. As we watched our kids go down the slide, I noticed she kept apologizing for her son, Colton, because he had pushed my daughter out of the way a few times so he could go down the slide first.

Becca apologized for interrupting our small talk, saying, "I don't want him to push your daughter. I'll be right back." She walked over to Colton and reminded him that everyone was entitled to their own turn. She reminded him not to push. She reminded him to use his words. Despite her being frazzled and full of apologies, I liked her immediately since she was doing what I had done in the past.

"I appreciate you helping him so the kids can take turns," I told her.

"I'm sorry he's so aggressive. He doesn't have many words yet."

"I get it," I replied. "You don't need to apologize. You're up there, helping him navigate this situation."

"I wish he wouldn't push. This has been happening a lot lately. I want him to wait patiently."

"He will—eventually. You're doing a great job with him."

Becca cracked a tiny smile, drew a deep breath, and whispered, "Thank you." I noticed her eyes filling with tears.

"Being a mom is exhausting, isn't it?" I said.

She wiped away a tear and nodded.

"All of us are doing the best that we can."

ACCEPTING AND EMBRACING DISABILITY

No one is perfect. I am *far* from perfect. Imperfection is part of the human condition.

When we scroll through social media, we are greeted with a curated version of other people's lives. Seeing a highlight reel is great, but life is rarely perfect. The competitive bragging we see on various platforms can sting when raising a child who isn't accomplishing as much as peers the same age.

As the parent of a child with multiple nonvisible disabilities (see the box on page 14), I often felt compressed in a narrow place when I scrolled through social media during the early years of my daughter's life. While other parents attended classes and discovered new playgrounds, I shuttled my daughter to speech, occupational, and physical therapies. I was exhausted. I sought help and answers as my daughter acquired new labels from medical professionals. I looked for a way to get to the other side . . . to a place that looked like the curated version of my Facebook friends' lives.

What If Your Child's Disability Isn't Visible to Others?

Nonvisible disabilities, often referred to as non-apparent disabilities, present differently in public than visible disabilities—they may not always be recognized by others in the same way as disabilities that require mobility aids or assistive technology. This often leaves you to find a way to help those in your child's social environment understand, and it's not always easy. I've learned over almost a decade how to navigate various domains of my child's life to promote respect and compassion—and I have helped her learn how to advocate for herself as she matures. I'll pass on what I've learned throughout this book.

Over time, I began sharing the less glamorous parts of our lives. I shared pictures from advocacy walks. I shared videos of my daughter as she acquired new words. In time, I shared about overcoming struggles as I watched my daughter become a reader. I shared these things on social media and my blogs, so other parents whose lives weren't perfectly curated would begin celebrating all parts of their children too.

As I mentioned in the Introduction, many people treat *disability* as a four-letter word. They try to replace it with terms like *special needs* or *differently abled*. This happens because many people think of disability as a negative thing . . . something wrong with someone. As parents of disabled children, we know our child's disability is part of who they are. It's part of our child's identity and isn't something to be ashamed of.

"One billion people, or 15% of the world's population, experience some form of disability," according to the World Bank Group. Sit with that for a moment. *One Billion People*. That is a significant minority group. As parents of disabled kids, we are not alone.

THE LANGUAGE OF DISABILITY

As a parent of a disabled child, you will hear a dizzying array of terms used to describe conditions that fall under the wide umbrella of disabilities. It's important to recognize that how disabilities are categorized depends on the purpose of the classification. The following is one way to conceptualize disabilities in a broad sense. As you'll see in Chapter 2, when schools formulate Individualized Education Programs (IEPs) for students, they use a different breakdown.

Types of Disabilities

Disabilities take many forms and affect individuals in unique ways. Below are broad categories that cover many common types, though individual experiences will vary and there is often some overlap.

- **Chronic medical conditions:** persistent, long-term health conditions that often lack a cure and continuously impact various aspects of a person's physical and mental well-being. Chronic medical conditions include asthma, Crohn's disease, diabetes, epilepsy, and multiple sclerosis.

- **Communication disorders:** trouble understanding, using, or processing different forms of communication. A communication disorder can affect someone's ability to hear, speak, or understand language. Communication disorders can vary in severity, from mild to very serious. They can be present at birth or develop later in life.

- **Developmental disabilities:** a group of conditions that can affect how a person's body, learning, language, or behavior develops. These conditions start during childhood and can continue throughout a person's life. They cause limitations in different areas because of problems with the developing nervous system. These limitations can manifest as delays in reaching milestones or difficulties in thinking, moving, seeing, hearing, talking, and/or behaving.

- **Hearing disabilities:** conditions in which an individual has a partial or complete inability to hear sounds. Hearing disabilities can range in severity from mild to profound. They can be present from birth or can happen later in life. Hearing disabilities can impact a person's ability to perceive, understand, and communicate through spoken language or other auditory cues.

- **Intellectual disabilities:** a developmental condition that can impact an individual's cognitive functioning and other skills, such as language, social interaction, and self-care. These limitations can lead to a slower or different development and learning trajectory than individuals without intellectual disabilities.

- **Learning disabilities:** disorders that impact how people learn, process, and comprehend subjects like reading, writing, and math. They can also hinder higher-level skills such as organization, time management, abstract reasoning, and memory (both short-term and long-term). These disabilities are rooted in biological differences. Heredity also plays a role, as learning disabilities often run in families. Importantly, learning disabilities are unrelated to intelligence, meaning they do not reflect a person's overall intellectual capabilities. Most learning disabilities do not resolve or disappear over time; individuals typically do not outgrow them.

- **Mental health disabilities:** various conditions that impact a person's thoughts, moods, and behavior. They refer to various mental health conditions such as anxiety, depression, obsessive-compulsive disorder, and post-traumatic stress disorder. These conditions affect cognition, mood, and behavior, leading to challenges in functioning and daily life activities.

- **Neurodevelopmental disorders:** conditions that affect how the brain develops, works, and processes. They can make it harder for people to learn, communicate, and interact with others. ADHD and autism are examples of neurodevelopmental disorders.

- **Neurological disorders:** conditions that impact various parts of a person's nervous system, including the brain, spinal cord, nerves throughout the body, and the autonomic nervous system. These disorders can affect individuals physically, cognitively, and emotionally. Examples of neurological disorders are epilepsy and migraines.

- **Physical disabilities:** impacts a person's ability to move, use their hands, or maintain stamina. These disabilities involve limitations or disabilities that restrict the function of one or more limbs. They can be temporary or permanent. Physical disabilities can arise from various causes, including inherited or genetic disorders, serious illnesses, or injuries.

- **Sensory processing disorders:** involve challenges in processing and responding to sensory information (such as movement, sound, or touch), leading to responses that can impact behavior and everyday functioning. Neurodivergent individuals, such as those with autism or ADHD, are often affected, sometimes being overwhelmed by sensory input, and other times not noticing it as much or being under-responsive.

- **Vision disabilities:** conditions that partially or entirely hinder a person's ability to see. Individuals with vision impairments have difficulties that regular glasses, contact lenses, medication, or surgery cannot correct. Even with glasses or contact lenses, they may encounter challenges in performing everyday tasks. Vision disabilities arise when an eye condition affects the visual system and its vision-related functions.

This list shows that some disabilities are visible while others are hidden. Some children have visible and nonvisible disabilities, while others have disabilities that are nonapparent to others as they go through life.

A year after we met on the playground, Becca recounted how she felt when filling out a form for medical assistance for Colton. There was a question asking her whether or not her child was disabled. She had to acknowledge Colton's disability if she wanted him to qualify for the secondary insurance she needed to pay for all of his medical expenses and therapies. Due to internalized ableism, she hesitated before checking the box to attest that Colton was disabled. However, acknowledging Colton's disability on that form was a salient moment. It helped her understand that her silly, handsome, and headstrong son had a disability . . . it was part of him.

It's essential to know that using the word *disability* will get your child the services, funding, and care they need. If calling autism a disability (see the box below) provides your children access to what they need, then put the word *disability* on it.

Are Neurodivergence and Neurodiversity Disabilities?

Neurodivergence and neurodiversity challenge the traditional view of disability. In *Against Technoableism: Rethinking Who Needs Improvement*, Ashley Shew explains that identifying as neurodivergent aligns with the disability community in that social norms and expectations can make neurodivergence disabling, just as different architectural designs can highlight physical disabilities. Shew clarifies that autistic individuals and those with ADHD originated the concepts of neurodivergence and neurodiversity, but the larger disability community has embraced them. Some people use neurodivergence to resist being labeled as disabled, while others see themselves as part of the disability community.

Disability Models

There are several lenses, known as *models*, for viewing disability. There are individualistic or deficit-based models, which include the charity model, the economic model, the medical model, and the moral model. In other words, disability is viewed as a deficiency, a weakness, or something to be fixed. Some models are asset-based, such as the human rights and social models of disability. Each model considers the perceived causes or origins of disability, the appropriate actions or responses to address disability, and the deeper meanings or implications associated with disability. The medical and social models are most frequently discussed in the literature and the ones you're most likely to encounter.

Medical Model of Disability

- Views disability as a problem in the body's systems or functions that is considered inherently abnormal or unhealthy
- Aims to bring the body's systems or functions back to a state considered "normal" or typical

- Expects individuals with disabilities to follow the advice of health care professionals
- Uses clinical and medical language within health care, mental health, and educational settings
- Perceives disability as an individual defect, emphasizing the need to cure or eliminate disabilities for a higher quality of life
- Notes that messages conveying low expectations and fear of disability can result in limited opportunities for individuals with disabilities

Social Model of Disability

- Acknowledges that disability is not the fault of the individual but a result of societal barriers
- Views disability as the result of how individuals interact with an environment that doesn't provide the necessary accommodations for their needs and differences
- Emphasizes the importance of removing societal barriers rather than fixing individuals
- Advocates for eliminating physical, social, and communication barriers to ensure full inclusion in the community
- Considers disability one aspect of a person's identity, similar to race or gender
- Believes the mismatch between the disabled person and the environment creates barriers
- Focuses on changing the environment and society rather than changing individuals
- Seeks to end discrimination against people with disabilities through education, accommodations, and barrier-free spaces
- Recognizes that eliminating disability would hinder the appreciation of diverse ways of being in the world

Most of us have beliefs that fall into more than one model. I believe the social model values disabled children for who they are and reflects the idea that we, as parents and society in general, must change to meet their needs.

Person-First Language versus Identity-First Language

Person-first language puts the person before their diagnosis, whereas identity-first language emphasizes a person's diagnosis first.

Person-First Language	Identity-First Language
Person with a Disability	Disabled Person
Person with Autism	Autistic Person
Person with Dyslexia	Dyslexic Person
Person with Visual Impairment	Visually Impaired Person

The disability community debates whether to use person-first or identity-first language. As the parent of a person with multiple nonvisible disabilities, I often use person-first language since it allows me to recognize my daughter, reaffirming her personhood rather than focusing on her disabilities. She vacillates between person-first and identity-first language, so I follow her lead.

People with disabilities usually prefer one term or another, so it's best to take a person-centered approach, asking the person how they choose to identify (for instance, "Do you prefer person- or identity-first language?"). Check the Resources at the end of this book for some articles on person-first versus identity-first language.

Knowing that many children in elementary school may not have a preference, this book will tend to use person-first language.

High-Functioning and Low-Functioning

High-functioning and low-functioning are insulting and flawed concepts. Neither of these labels is a compliment. The way someone functions can vary from day to day and year to year. Furthermore, these labels pit people with disabilities against each other regarding accessing the support they need. In *Demystifying Disability: What to Know, What to Say, and How to Be an Ally*, Emily Ladau suggests:

> Consider a conversation between a parent of a young child with a disability and the child's teacher. Rather than referring to the student as "low functioning" in math, the teacher can say, "I've noticed your child needs more support in completing his math assignments" or "Your child might benefit from extra support to complete her math homework." Such language is simple, straightforward, and respectful without placing a harmful label on the student.

THINKING ABOUT STRENGTHS

How do you talk about your child when someone asks about them? Do you lead with their strengths or weaknesses? Do you talk about their successes or their struggles? Do you label them?

Here's an example of how I talk about my daughter, who sparked the idea for this book:

> "My child is 14. She's highly organized, motivated to complete her schoolwork on time or ahead of schedule, and works diligently to achieve good grades. She has a gorgeous singing voice and sings in her school's chorus. She learned another language at a young age and continues to study it. She loves the water and participates on a summer swim team. She probably swims nearly a mile during every practice! She doesn't complain when she has to dive into a chilly pool when her coach gives directions. My daughter is a caring older sister who loves her little brother. Even though he bugs her often, she thinks of him as her best friend."

Describing a child's strengths is essential since it positions them positively. No one is perfect. Not the high school valedictorian or the quarterback of the football team. Since many people would not lead with a nondisabled person's flaws, *we shouldn't talk about a disabled person by what they cannot do.* We should see the whole child and talk about the fantastic things that person *can* do.

Let's be honest. *Everyone* has needs. There's nothing special about them. You will see the phrase *higher support needs*, but you won't see the term *special needs* used in this book.

ELIMINATING DEFICIT-BASED LABELS IN SCHOOL

Over the years, many well-meaning teachers have used deficit-based labels when discussing children. For instance, they might say, "Kylie is a struggling writer" or "Joe is below grade level as a reader." Instead of doing this, it's essential to talk about what a child needs to grow. It's crucial to adopt language that is individualized and actionable. The language should put the onus on adults at all levels—from the classroom to the school district office—so we can provide children with what they need to grow.

I'm on a family advisory committee in our school district. This is a small group of parents (whose children have IEPs) who meet with the director of special education quarterly. One thing I've proposed is using more inclusive language. For example, *general education* instead of regular *education* (also, *higher support needs* instead of *lower functioning*). Six months after proposing the idea, the director reported working with her staff to be more intentional with their words in meetings, on paperwork, and about students.

Adult language should start with strength and then name the actionable teaching to provide the next step. Here are two strength-based examples that put the child's strength first and then explain what they'll need to grow:

- Kylie will use her public speaking skills to lead her peers in a writing process share session in three monthly end-of-workshop share sessions.
- Given third-grade level nonfiction reading material, Joe will deploy his interest in social studies to write three details from the passage in his own words with 85% accuracy on three out of four consecutive assignments.

Melanie Meehan discussed the language used to talk about students with high needs. In *Every Child Can Write: Entry Points, Bridges and Pathways for Striving Writers*, Melanie wrote, "While I grapple with *any* term, striving implies effort, and I want to believe that everyone is wired and willing to *try*; people don't *choose* to struggle." Let's remove references like *struggling writers* and *low reading levels* from our conversations about kids. We can shift our language so we're positioning students in a way that ensures they're striving to do their personal best.

ON TO THE EVALUATION PROCESS

With the foundation you've established in this chapter, you're prepared to dive into the evaluation process. The next chapter focuses on trusting your gut (since you are your child's first teacher) when it comes to getting your child evaluated in an educational setting.

———————————————

In fifth grade, Colton invited a friend over to their house for a play date. The boys were still playing in the backyard when the other child's mother arrived to pick him up. Becca invited her to sit on their patio while the boys kicked soccer balls around in the backyard.

Becca had only met this boy's mother once before but fell into an easy conversation about their wonderful sons, both of whom faced challenges. The other mom casually mentioned her son's intellectual and mental health disability in the conversation. Becca shared one of Colton's early diagnoses relevant to their discussion about how school was going. She didn't flinch when Becca mentioned Colton's challenges, and Becca didn't blink when she told Colton's mom about her son's disabilities.

After they parted, Becca texted me about the conversation. "Seven years ago, when we met on that playground, I never would have shared Colton's diagnosis with a virtual stranger." Information like that was held close by her and was shared only with people she could trust. But her mindset had changed since she'd applied for medical assistance years earlier. Becca understood Colton's disabilities were one part of who he is. There was no shame in talking about them! Communicating openly with others about who our children are— their strengths and their challenges—normalizes disability.

Tip for Cultivating Joy: Use social media mindfully. While social media is a fantastic way to stay in touch with friends and family, it can also make you feel down. Reduce your use of social media platforms that leave you feeling disheartened.

Self-Care Tip: Slowing your breathing down is one way to manage stressful situations. Rather than waiting for stressful moments, practice slow breathing techniques now! Extended exhalations are associated with slowing the heart rate, which lessens the stress response. (You can read about this at *www.psychologytoday.com/us /blog/the-athletes-way/201905/longer-exhalations-are-easy-way-hack -your-vagus-nerve*.) While I'm partial to using longer outbreaths and Box Breathing to decrease my stress level, it's essential to find breathing exercises that work for you. (See Self-Care Resources.) Practice one or two breathing exercises for a few minutes daily so they're well-practiced and ready to be activated when you are stressed.

2

Chart Your Course through the Evaluation Process

Aiden's occupational therapist came out to talk with his mom, Rachel, at the end of every appointment. In mid-May, she said gravely, "Do you have a few minutes?"

Rachel braced herself. What kind of news was she going to receive now?

The OT was straightforward when she told Rachel that she was concerned Aiden could be dysgraphic.

After asking the OT to explain dysgraphia, Rachel asked, "Can you do that testing?"

"I can't test and diagnose, but the school district can do educational testing," she replied.

"But Aiden attends private school," she retorted.

"You're still entitled to an evaluation from your local public school since you're a taxpayer," the OT asserted.

"I am?"

(Rachel had been used to having all of Aiden's testing done at a hospital-based facility where she took her son for his therapies.)

"You are. It doesn't matter that Aiden doesn't attend public elementary school. The local elementary school will have its school psychologist administer some testing. You will have to submit a letter and must be specific about your concerns when requesting the evaluation."

Rachel's eyes welled with tears. More. Testing.

"Write a letter as soon as possible and hand-deliver it to the school," the OT instructed. "It's almost summer break. You'll want them to have that letter ASAP since the clock starts running as soon as they have your evaluation request letter. They have to send you a Permission to Evaluate-Consent form. From there, they have 60 calendar days to evaluate Aiden once they receive the signed form. However, in our state, summer calendar days do not count."

This was going to take a while.

Rachel crafted a letter requesting an evaluation in late May. In the letter, she stated her son's past diagnoses and included copies of all testing results. She thought sharing documentation from previous testing and her concerns would be helpful. Rachel hand-delivered the letter to the public elementary school on May 24. Testing began in early September. However, Rachel didn't meet to review the evaluation report until November 1.

Rachel was frustrated at the meeting since the testing wasn't complete when the IEP team met on November 1. She wondered how it was possible that the school district's school psychologist had completed the testing, but the occupational therapist still had a couple more tests that needed to be administered. The occupational therapist didn't complete the testing until late November. Rachel was frustrated further when Aiden's IEP adoption meeting didn't happen until mid-January.

REQUESTING A COMPREHENSIVE SCHOOL-BASED EDUCATIONAL EVALUATION

As a parent, you know your child best. Your child might struggle academically, behaviorally, emotionally, or socially at school. In that case, your right as a parent is to request an evaluation to determine whether they have a disability and qualify for specialized instruction, related services, or other supports.

My friend once described the evaluation process as looking for the key to unlock a child's brain so they could find an easier path to learning and living. That is the most beautiful way to describe *why* we try to determine what's impacting our child. I love this mindset because all parents want their children to have an easier life and an easier time in school.

> Think of an evaluation as looking for the key to unlock your child's brain so they can find an easier path to learning and living.

Contacting your child's teacher before requesting an evaluation is vital since there are many options before a school-based evaluation. You can request a face-to-face meeting, even if an IEP isn't in place. There's a lot of value in conferring like this. The school needs to understand what you're noticing at home. Likewise, they can give you a better perspective on your child's school life. During the meeting, you can review work samples, assessments, and screeners to determine the next steps and whether more intervention is needed.

Common Interventions

MTSS, or Multi-Tiered System of Supports, is an educational, schoolwide framework designed to provide support and extra help to students who are not meeting benchmarks. It has different academic, behavioral, and social-emotional supports based on students' needs. Tier 1 focuses on high-quality instruction for the whole class. Tier 2 provides targeted interventions for individuals who require additional support, typically conducted in small groups. Tier 3 provides intensive support for students who require additional assistance, either individually or in small groups. Students who don't progress with Tier 3 interventions often get referred for a special education evaluation. MTSS uses data (often referred to as *assessment and progress monitoring*) to make informed decisions, relies on research-based practices, and encourages collaboration between teachers, administrators, and parents to help students succeed.

MTSS is a holistic approach that evolved from the integration of positive behavioral interventions and supports (PBIS) and response to intervention (RTI) to ensure that all students have access to effective, high-quality instruction. It is comprehensive because it includes academic, behavioral, and social-emotional pieces. If you think of MTSS as an umbrella, PBIS and RTI fall under the MTSS umbrella.

Schools have implemented various systems and terms over the years, with different acronyms. However, it's important to note that a child's pathway to special education often involves increasingly specialized instruction that doesn't necessarily accelerate their learning curve as intended. Despite tiered interventions, some students face persistent roadblocks that cause their achievement gap to widen rather than close. This ongoing challenge highlights the complexity of addressing diverse learning needs and the importance of continually refining and improving support systems within the MTSS framework.

- **PBIS** is an approach that helps create a positive and supportive school environment for students. It focuses on teaching and reinforcing good behavior rather than just punishing misbehavior. Tier 1 offers universal support promoting positive behavior for all students. It includes teaching and reinforcing clear expectations, rules, and routines regularly. Students receive praise, recognition, and rewards for demonstrating positive behavior. Tier 2 offers targeted support and interventions to support students who need extra assistance in meeting behavioral expectations. Small-group interventions, social skills training, or mentoring programs address specific behavioral needs. In Tier 3, students struggling with behavior receive more intensive interventions, such as individualized behavior plans, counseling, or additional support from specialists. By focusing on positive reinforcement and providing necessary support, PBIS aims to prevent problem behaviors, improve student well-being, and enhance academic success for all students.

- **RTI** is an approach that helps students struggling with academics or at risk of falling behind. It involves three tiers of support. With RTI, teachers assess using tests and observations to identify students who need extra support. Next, identified students receive targeted interventions based on their needs. Interventions occur through small-group instruction, one-on-one tutoring, or specialized programs. Finally, teachers regularly monitor students' progress to see whether the interventions work. They adjust the support if needed to meet the student's needs better. RTI aims to catch problems early, provide timely support, and ensure all students can succeed.

Once extra support has been implemented, it's wise to check in with the classroom teacher to see how your child has responded to interventions and informal accommodations. If your child has not made progress after some time has passed since implementing interventions, and you suspect they may have a disability, I recommend that you request an evaluation. You need to be the squeaky wheel if your child isn't closing the gap with the provided interventions. Sometimes, schools don't have the same sense of urgency when determining if your child is progressing, so it's up to you to nudge things along.

The Evaluation Process

The evaluation process may seem overwhelming, but it is manageable. I'm going to help you understand what to expect and how to proceed.

Begin by having a conversation with the principal or the special education department. Explain your concerns and get informed about the next steps, the timeline in your state (how many days it will take to begin an evaluation and how long the district has to complete it), decision-making procedures, etc. After that conversation, you may submit a written request to have your child evaluated, which also provides written documentation of the discussion.

When submitting a written request for a comprehensive educational evaluation, you'll want to briefly tell the story of your child's history and why you wish to receive a special education evaluation (see the box on pages 29–30 for a list of disabilities that qualify). Explaining your suspicions about a disability and other concerns in writing can help the school psychologist understand the assessments needed to determine your child's strengths and needs.

An evaluation team at your child's school will meet to decide if there's a preponderance of evidence that your child could have a disability. This team may include your child's teacher, a school psychologist, an administrator, and relevant specialists (such as a speech therapist). The evaluation team will likely review various sources of information, such as assessments, observations, and reports, to gather evidence regarding your child's developmental, academic, and behavioral functioning. They will consider this evidence collectively to determine the next steps they will take.

You will probably initiate your own evaluation requests, but be aware that IDEA requires LEAs to actively locate, identify, and evaluate all children from birth through age 21 living in their jurisdiction who may have disabilities and need special education services. This legal requirement is known as Child Find, and it applies to children even if they are not enrolled in public school, are homeschooled, or attend private school.

Who Qualifies for Special Education?

The Individuals with Disabilities Education Act (IDEA) mandates that public schools give eligible students special education and related services. However, not all children who have difficulties in school qualify for these services. To be eligible, *a child's educational performance must be adversely affected* by a disability in one of these 13 categories:

1. Autism
2. Deaf-blindness
3. Deafness
4. Emotional Disturbance
5. Hearing Impairment
6. Intellectual Disability
7. Multiple Disabilities
8. Orthopedic Impairment
9. Other Health Impairment
10. Specific Learning Disability
11. Speech or Language Impairment
12. Traumatic Brain Injury
13. Visual Impairment, including blindness

Prior Written Notice is a way for schools to communicate with parents about any actions they plan to take or not take regarding their child. Parents must be well informed about what the school is proposing—or *refusing* to do (see the box on pages 29–30). By providing Prior Written Notice, the school ensures parents understand the school's proposed actions or their refusal to evaluate a child.

Why Would a School Deny a Request for an Evaluation?

It is within the school's right to deny a special education evaluation if it believes there is no evidence of a disability. Some common reasons for denial are as follows:

- The child started school recently (kindergarten, first grade), and the school believes they will catch up with developmental milestones.
- The child's grades are improving through interventions that the school is already providing.
- The child's impairment does not substantially limit major life activities related to school.
- The child is an EAL (English as an Additional Language) student, and the school feels additional language instruction is needed instead of special education.
- The child's struggles are attributed to willful behavior rather than an underlying issue.

The school must explain its decision to deny an evaluation in writing. You may call a meeting to discuss further the detailed reasons for the denial, including a request for data that informed the decision. If you disagree with the school's decision after the meeting, you can have your child evaluated independently or take steps to overturn the school's decision.

An evaluation plan is created if the school proceeds with a special education evaluation. The school psychologist works to determine whether or not your child has a disability. Before beginning testing, they will confer with you to get more information about your child. Gathering information from you may include rating scales, checklists, and live conversations to learn more about how your child functions at home, your academic/behavioral/social concerns, etc. The school psychologist may observe your child during the school day to understand how your child functions in the classroom, during related arts periods, at lunch, or on the playground. Most importantly, the school psychologist administers a variety of assessments.

The areas a school psychologist will evaluate will guide the tools (academic, behavioral, cognitive, psychological assessment, etc.) they use. To help them choose the proper assessments and rating scales, you can do a few things to make their job easier:

- Fill out forms and rating scales accurately and return them promptly.
- Send over accompanying medical information from your child's providers as soon as possible.

- Provide any evaluation reports you have from outside evaluators. External evaluations help support the school-based evaluation and help the school psychologist determine what assessments have been done so they are not repeated.

More testing isn't always better. Think about it like this: When someone comes to the emergency room with an injury, some get an X-ray while others get an MRI. The physician determines what tests to do based on the patient's presentation. It's the same thing with the testing that happens during an evaluation. School psychologists review the data and input from parents and teachers to determine the most suitable tests to administer. Sometimes, less testing is better, as kids can become exhausted from excessive testing over several weeks.

FIVE THINGS TO DO DURING THE EVALUATION PROCESS

- Respect the timing. You need to give the school the number of days—typically 45–60 days—your state mandates to complete the evaluation.
- Be patient. You can check in with the school, but don't rush the evaluation. Your child isn't the only student who needs to be evaluated. Plus, once the testing begins, it takes time for the evaluators to gather data, carry out the testing, and interpret the results.
- Explain to your child. Please help your child understand that the testing will take time and might mean they have to miss parts of their school day, but it will help their teachers make learning and living easier.
- Make sure your child is present. Communicate with evaluators if your child will be absent for a medical appointment or religious reason during the evaluation period. Ensure your child has had as much sleep as possible, has eaten a healthy breakfast, and has taken their medication (if applicable) before testing so they can do their personal best.
- Communicate with the teacher. Ensure your child receives as much teacher support, interventions, and accommodations as possible during the testing. Be sure to express appreciation, since this fosters a positive relationship.

Once the evaluation process is finished, a written report is prepared. In this report, the school psychologist and any other evaluators involved in the evaluation write about their specific findings and observations. The report includes the reasons for the evaluation request and any relevant scores or measurements obtained during the evaluation. In addition, the report provides a summary of what the evaluators have learned about the child's abilities and needs based on the evaluation.

Next, if a student qualifies for special education, an eligibility meeting is scheduled with the evaluators and the IEP team members at a mutually agreeable time. The evaluation report must be shared with you before the meeting so you can review it and jot down any questions. The evaluators will present their results and recommendations at the eligibility meeting and determine if your child needs an IEP.

The school team will create an IEP if your child meets the eligibility criteria under one of the 13 disability designations outlined by IDEA. The criteria for some of these disabilities (specific learning disability criteria, for one) may differ from state to state or district to district. It is crucial to grasp the eligibility criteria used in your state or district. The school psychologist should be able to explain them. Typically, within 30 calendar days, the IEP team must meet to develop the child's IEP.

The IEP team includes the following:

- Parent
- Representative of the public agency (such as principal, special education director)
- Special education teacher
- General education teacher

The IEP team may also include the following:

- Additional teachers
- Counselor
- Related service providers (OT, PT, speech)

An IEP will serve as a contract listing your child's goals (such as that, in a 12-month period, your child is expected to learn or do certain things) and the services they'll provide to help them meet each goal. Your consent is required before special education programs and services can be provided to your child for the first time. Once your written consent is given, the IEP must be implemented within about 10 school days. However, check with your state's PTI or education department to ensure you know your state's IEP implementation guidelines. For instance, at the time of writing, Texas required five school days, whereas Oregon required 10 school days to implement an IEP.

Honoring Your Intuition

Rachel recounted that she stared in disbelief when she received Aiden's evaluation report. It said: "The student has a disability AND is in need of specially designed instruction, and therefore is eligible for special education." His primary disability category was "specific learning disability related to listening comprehension." No secondary or tertiary disabilities were identified, despite Aiden carrying an ADHD diagnosis from his developmental pediatrician.

Rachel wondered how the school psychologist could think Aiden's needs were related only to listening comprehension and long-term memory retrieval. Nothing concerning was mentioned about reading, writing, or math. Rachel was flummoxed that the assessment didn't adequately reflect the difficulties she observed at home.

After scouring through the testing results and written observations by the school district's evaluators, Rachel attended the eligibility meeting with numerous questions. The folks in the meeting explained how the testing had informed the disability category they gave Aiden. Still, they could not answer her questions about how they'd help Aiden overcome the challenges they noted with listening comprehension and long-term memory retrieval. Everything was fuzzy. Rachel worried the IEP team wouldn't be able to help Aiden progress since they couldn't articulate what was next.

While waiting for an IEP adoption meeting, Rachel consulted nearly every professional she knew in child development and education. She wanted to know what they thought a "specific learning disability related to listening comprehension" was and how they would help Aiden. Professional after professional was bewildered, considering the concerns about dysgraphia and Aiden's existing ADHD diagnosis. This designation made sense to anyone who knew Aiden and his struggles.

Due to Aiden's enrollment in a private school and the need for daily bus rides to the public school for specialized listening disorder instruction, Rachel requested that his IEP be implemented at the start of the following school year. Rachel didn't want to pay private school tuition and have her son miss out on 90 or more minutes of his school day to get services for a disability he might not have.

Knowing that Aiden sometimes had inconsistent attention due to his ADHD diagnosis, Rachel's gut told her the school district's testing had missed the mark. Rachel knew she needed to have Aiden evaluated privately by a neuropsychologist, who could ascertain what was happening with him. And it needed to happen fast!

Private Evaluations

Rania had a school-based evaluation that revealed a specific learning disability. In addition, the school psychologist noted that Rania had executive functioning issues. The IEP team did not schedule Rania to receive any support for her executive functioning deficits, even though these deficits were noted during in-class observations and testing. Rania's parents wanted additional information to help her at home and school. They visited a neuropsychologist who assessed her executive functioning by learning more about Rania's attention, working memory, and visual-spatial skills. The neuropsychologist determined what the deficit was and provided Rania's parents with recommendations to improve Rania's time management, organization, and problem-solving skills at home. In addition, the neuropsychologist included recommendations for Rania's teacher to implement at school to help Rania improve her executive functioning there. Thankfully, Rania's school was receptive to the suggestions provided by the neuropsychologist. Her case manager was willing to include several recommendations as specially designed instruction in Rania's IEP.

Rania's parents felt it was worth the time and expense (see more about costs—admittedly often high—later in this chapter) to hire an outside neuropsychologist to conduct additional assessments because they felt Rania was struggling with things her older siblings didn't have issues with when they were Rania's age. They were unsure what they could do to help Rania get more organized, be less impulsive, and better manage her time so they wouldn't have to micromanage her at home. While seeking outside help was time-consuming and expensive, they were thankful they could learn more about how

Rania's brain worked so she could become more goal-directed and self-regulated.

Most school districts thoroughly administer testing and convey the results of school-based evaluations. They have well-trained staff members who do an excellent job communicating with families and helping teachers understand a child's needs so they can thrive at school with the right help. Rachel got unlucky when she had Aiden's initial school-based evaluation done. Is she glad it happened? Nope. Is Aiden better off *now* because his parents sought a second opinion to determine the root cause of his academic troubles? Absolutely.

I encourage you to seek out a more comprehensive evaluation if you want more specific answers about your child's disability or feel unsure about the results of a school-based evaluation. Additional assessments can provide valuable insights into your child's strengths and challenges.

Rachel and her husband, Brent, met with a neuropsychologist in February. They shared the school-based evaluation with her and explained that it confounded them. Both had a gut feeling that Aiden didn't have a listening comprehension disability. During the interview, the neuropsychologist spoke with Brent and Rachel at length so she could understand Aiden's challenges. Then she had them fill out multiple rating scales. Next came the testing, done over several weeks so Aiden didn't miss that much school. The neuropsychologist administered assessments to determine the following:

- Academic achievement
- Attention and working memory
- Executive functioning
- Fluid reasoning skills
- Intellectual ability
- Learning and memory
- Motor abilities
- Social perception
- Verbal skills
- Visual-spatial and visuomotor skills

By late April, Rachel and Brent received a detailed report explaining each test, what the child must do, the tasks assessed, scores, percentile rankings, and performance range. For the achievement tests, they also received the grade equivalency of each score. While reading the report overwhelmed them, the neuropsychologist met with them to explain the results, answer their questions, and share her recommendations.

Aiden's parents received abundant insight into Aiden's mind and how he would learn best in school. Aiden was diagnosed with a specific learning disorder with impairment in reading and a specific learning disorder with impairment in mathematics. The neuropsychologist also reconfirmed Aiden's ADHD diagnosis. They also learned the following, which came directly from the neuropsychologist's report:

"In the past, Aiden has been identified as a student with a disability in listening comprehension. However, in this evaluation, his verbal memory task performance, which requires listening comprehension, was average. It is suspected that past listening comprehension difficulties were the result of poor or inconsistent attention. When Aiden is focused, he is average in his ability to listen, understand, learn, and retain information outside of his areas of learning disability."

The neuropsychologist saw signs of dysgraphia but wasn't ready to diagnose Aiden with it. As a result, she encouraged Rachel and Brent to return in a couple of years if they had ongoing suspicions about dysgraphia.

This is what Rachel thought of as a mic drop moment! Rachel was delighted that her child had average listening abilities, despite having ADHD. It shows that Rachel's hunch about Aiden was right because she knew her son best.

Questioning and Seeking Additional Opinions

What everyone should know as they go through the evaluation process is that you can request an independent educational evaluation, or IEE, from their school district.

Independent Educational Evaluations

Under the IDEA, parents have the legal right to request an IEE if they disagree with the results of a school-based evaluation, think it wasn't thorough enough, or it didn't find evidence of a disability. The school district may have to pay for an IEE if the parent doesn't agree with the testing or if the testing isn't considered thorough enough. However, a school district won't just give away IEEs to every family that asks for one. Given that public resources fund it, you must proactively seek an IEE and provide compelling evidence to support your child's need for this evaluation. You may also decide to seek the help of an advocate; see the box below.

Are you worried about being labeled as "difficult" or "overly concerned" if you request an IEE? It is a valid concern. But remember, you are advocating for your child's needs. If you respectfully express your concerns about the school-based evaluation results, you are more likely to be labeled an "advocate" for your child, which is good!

Do You Need an Advocate?

You can seek an advocate to help you if you need additional support. These professionals understand the IEP process and the special education system and can help you as you work to meet your child's needs. If you meet with one, however, you should ask what training and experience they have and what their plan is for your child. There are free and low-cost advocates, while some advocates charge a few hundred dollars per hour. Start with your statewide Parent Center (mentioned in the Introduction) since they'll know your state's Protection and Advocacy Systems, or P&As. In addition, Parent Centers maintain lists of advocates with proper training. You may also access the member directory from the Council of Parent Attorneys and Advocates, or COPAA. They also have a detailed list of guidelines to help you choose an advocate.

If the school district agrees to pay for an IEE, they'll provide a list of providers not employed by your school system, so you can choose who will complete the IEE. The school district might offer to pay a specific amount to cover the IEE—whatever is consistent with what independent evaluators in your geographic area charge.

A school must consider the IEE, or any private evaluation's findings, when deciding how to educate your child. However, the school is not required to agree with the IEE or follow its recommendations. The school must base its decision on providing your child with a free and appropriate public education (FAPE).

A school has the right to challenge your request for an IEE, which could mean you will end up in a due process hearing where a due process hearing officer, who is a neutral third party, examines your request and the school's objection. If you can provide enough evidence that the school-based evaluation wasn't enough or was inaccurate, the hearing officer can order the school district to pay for an IEE. But if the hearing officer decides the school's evaluation was correct, you'll have to pay for any independent evaluation you choose to pursue.

> **TIP** It's important to explain what you want for your child, aiming to minimize drama while making it clear that you understand how to escalate matters if necessary. Bottom line: You don't want to seem like you want to go to a due process hearing or even to court.

Finding an External Evaluator

You may decide to have your child evaluated privately *before* requesting a school-based evaluation, or you may choose not to go down the IEE path. You may hire an external evaluator to determine whether your child has a disability. Four types of private, independent practitioners can administer testing. Who you choose depends on what you want to know about your child.

- A **clinical child psychologist** helps children with mental health issues, like anxiety, behavioral issues, or depression. This professional can administer mental health testing and coordinate your child's care with your child's physician or a child psychiatrist.

- An **educational psychologist**'s primary role is to evaluate and diagnose learning difficulties, developmental delays, behavioral issues, and emotional challenges that may impact a person's academic progress. These psychologists may also provide additional services such as collaborating with a school, therapeutic counseling, and other forms of guidance.

- **Neuropsychologists** administer special tests to see how a child's brain is working when they exhibit attention, focus, and learning issues. These tests help make a plan to help the child learn and/or behave better. They can administer assessments that some school psychologists cannot give due to additional training. A neuropsychologist's evaluation and recommendations can serve as documentation to get your child accommodations in school.

- A private practice **school psychologist** operates independently to provide personalized assessment, intervention, and counseling services to students outside of a school environment.

Who Will Pay for an External Evaluator?

In some cases, medical insurance will pay for an evaluation. Some insurance might pay for ADHD or autism testing. However, medical insurance often covers only testing expenses leading to a medical diagnosis. Typically, it does not fund achievement assessments.

Paying for a private evaluation can be costly. Generally, you can expect to spend $3,000 to $7,000 for testing. It could cost more in areas like Chicago, New York City, and San Francisco, which have high living costs. Obtain cost estimates from evaluators regarding the approximate testing costs, considering the specific issues you want your child assessed. Be sure to ask if there are any additional fees.

There are lower or no-cost options available that can defray the cost of testing. Here are some things you can look into:

- Learning Disabilities Association of America, or LDA: LDA's website lists low-cost evaluation options. Visit *https://ldaamerica.org/support/state -affiliates* to find your local LDA office that can assist you in finding some in your region.

- National Alliance for Mental Health, or NAMI: You may contact the NAMI HelpLine or your local NAMI affiliate. Local affiliates have more local information and resources than the HelpLine. However, the HelpLine does have many national resources that may be useful. You may call to speak with a volunteer Information & Resource Referral Specialist by calling the NAMI HelpLine at 800-950-NAMI (6264), texting to 62640, or visiting *www.nami.org/help* to web chat with them.

- Parent Training and Information Center, or PTI: As mentioned in Chapter 1, there is at least one PTI in each state. They can help you find a lower or no-cost evaluator in your state. Visit *www.parentcenterhub.org/find-your-center* to find your local center.

- University-Based Testing Clinics: Many universities provide lower or no-cost options for learning disability or ADHD testing. Graduate students in psychology programs administer these tests under the guidance and supervision of an experienced psychologist. Some of these programs offer a sliding scale or payment plan if there's a fee involved in the testing. You can search online for "low-cost learning disability testing university" or see the Resources at the back of the book.

If you go the private route, share the results of an external evaluation with your child's school. The results will help them consider another professional's opinion and may help develop a more appropriate educational plan for your child.

> **TIP** Remember, school districts can do well on most evaluations. Always start by going through your school first. Once you go through the evaluation process, you can go the private route or seek an IEE if you can explain why the school-based evaluation fell short.

Cultivating Strong Partnerships during the Evaluation Process

For parents, the evaluation is highly personal. In the amount of time the law provides, the team working to evaluate your child is following the law and trying to help you determine whether your child has a disability. Some of these people will likely be working with your child for a year or more, so it's essential to be transparent about your child's needs and what you see at home from the start. There should be no secrets, because the educators working with you understand that you're advocating for your baby (even if your baby is in fifth grade and is almost as tall as you, they're still your baby!). Open communication from the beginning will allow you to cultivate relationships, leading to respectful communication, increased support, and a more collaborative approach to addressing your child's needs once the evaluation process is over.

Remember, during your child's evaluation timeline, the school psychologist and other evaluators may be evaluating several other children, plus providing services to students. They are busy. Rather than cold calling with a question or concern, I've found it helpful to find a mutually convenient time to speak on the phone via email, which sometimes means I'm talking to a teacher during their prep period or before or after-school hours. Even when the times given to me are less than ideal, I always strive to adjust my schedule to show my respect for the time commitments of others.

Bottom line, several things will help you through this process:

- **Collaboration is essential.** Feel free to ask questions if you are uncertain about your child's assessment scores, the assessment process, or the provided recommendations. Also, be available to answer any questions, even about your child's newborn and toddler years. There is no room for prioritizing privacy or withholding information if you want the evaluators to help your child.

- **Seek mutual understanding.** Ask questions if you don't understand what's happening during the process, the representation of your child's assessment scores, or the recommendations provided. It's okay if you don't understand and need time to process the information. It's hard to ask for more time given the time constraints of the IEP team, but it's always better to schedule an informal follow-up meeting if you need help synthesizing the information. In addition, if you think more time is needed for the IEP team to understand your child, you may communicate more via email.

- **Express gratitude.** Remember to say *thank you*, even if you feel frustrated. Showing gratitude, rather than being adversarial, goes a long way. The school is taking care of your child during the school day. Showing your thanks for the work educators do means a lot. Two ways to do this:
  - You can write handwritten notes or send thoughtful emails to express your appreciation for the time and effort the team is putting into your child.

o Take snacks to your child's IEP meeting. Bringing baked goods to an IEP meeting is a small gesture to show the team you appreciate their time and want to keep them nourished while they help you and your child.

- **Focus on a positive partnership**. No decisions can be made without you unless multiple attempts are made to involve you (and you don't show up). You are a part of the team! It should never be you *against* the school. Ensure that your actions and communications with the school say: *I want to be an active part of my child's IEP team. I want to work with you.*

- **Trust the process**. This is not the IEP team's first rodeo. These are professionals who understand the law and what they need to do to determine whether or not your child has a disability.

Aiden's parents were unable to obtain the necessary learning support for Aiden at his private school. Since they lost confidence in their local school district during the IEP evaluation process, they moved to a neighboring school district the following summer.

They had trepidations about sending Aiden to a public school with 500 students since he was used to a school with 200 kids, K–6. They worried he'd get lost in the crowd, have a horrible first day, and wouldn't want to return.

Yet when Rachel dropped Aiden off for the first day of school, the principal stood outside with several teachers and greeted Aiden warmly. The principal escorted Aiden into the building since they knew he might be nervous about where to go on his first day. Rachel was astounded by the warm welcome. It was the beginning of what turned out to be a successful school year for Aiden—both academically and socially.

INTUITION PLUS RESPECT

As you navigate the evaluation process, trust your intuition when you advocate for your child. If your child struggles, remember you don't have to navigate their challenges alone. Your local public school district is there to help!

From the moment you reach out to the school, engage in respectful communication. Remember that educators are overworked and trying to do right by every child, so it pays to respect everyone's time. Through your communication, be respectful to the institution while you advocate for your child's needs. Even if you seek a second opinion through an outside evaluator, communicate why and the results you receive directly and respectfully. School officials will look more favorably at any external testing results if they know why you sought external help. (Bottom line: It's to ensure you know as much as possible about your child so that they can thrive in school.) Remember, the people who work in schools are your allies, not your adversaries.

―――――――――――

Heather, a parent I had "met" through my blog, texted me because she was overwhelmed after taking her son for an external evaluation by a neuropsychologist. There was a diagnosis she expected, ADHD, but then there were other mental health disabilities piled on top of it, plus a specific learning disability. She was sitting in her office, going down an internet rabbit hole with her Google MD, trying to understand everything.

I texted back:

I'm glad you outsourced the testing and got the answers you sought, even if you learned more than expected. That's going to help you help David.

Remember, disability is one way of being human. David doesn't need to be cured or fixed, even if it feels like that's what you're being told.

You will get through this, and I'll be here to chat if you want to discuss things.

―――――――――――

Tip for Cultivating Joy: Play with your child, even if it's for 10 minutes each day, during the evaluation process. Allow your child to direct and pace the play so they're having fun alongside you. Visit the National Institute for Play's website to determine what kind of play is for you. (See Resources.) Then commit to playing daily. Even when demands are high and time is short, getting down to your child's level and engaging in play will bring more joy into your daily life.

Self-Care Tip: Filling out rating scales and profiles for evaluators can be tedious and time-consuming. Dedicate a fixed period each day for filling out forms. Stop when your timer goes off. While it's essential to return these items promptly, trying to complete everything in one to two days can lead to resentment of the process, so pace yourself.

Part II

Navigating the Education Maze

Maximizing Your Child's Education

3

Become Familiar
with the Landscape

I've been on both sides of an IEP meeting, first as a teacher and now as a parent. As a teacher, I presented information about how a student was progressing. Did I try to obtain additional services and supports to help my students succeed? Absolutely. But, at the end of the day, they were my student for one year. Once late June arrived, they would be someone else's responsibility.

There's a more considerable emotional investment when one is part of an IEP team in the parent role. Anytime I attend an IEP meeting, every person in the room introduces themselves by name and states their job title. It's whip-fast, so I jot down names and titles if someone I don't know is in the room. Typically, case managers ask if there are any parent concerns. Otherwise, it's a deep dive into an IEP of about 40–50 pages long! There is usually a time constraint since meetings occur before or during the school day. Being in the parent chair at an IEP meeting can feel overwhelming. Chapter 2 helped you understand the path you're likely to follow to get a useful evaluation of your child. However, it also helps to have a working knowledge of the landscape's features. This knowledge can keep you from getting stalled or taking unnecessary detours.

Whenever I visit a museum or an art gallery, I chat with docents to ask them where the special exhibitions are, what would be best given who I'm with (usually my kids), and so forth. These places are usually designed with specific themes or layouts, so knowing how to get the most out of the experience and maximize your time before you begin is crucial. Think of this chapter as a way to gain insight into the world of special education so that you understand the fundamentals before you explore further.

WHAT ARE RELATED SERVICES?

IDEA Section 300.34 provides a list of related services a child with an IEP can receive to help them access their public education program. The list includes the following:

1. Audiology
2. Counseling services
3. Early identification and assessment of disabilities in children
4. Interpreting services
5. Medical services
6. Occupational therapy
7. Orientation and mobility services
8. Parent counseling and training
9. Physical therapy
10. Psychological services
11. Recreation
12. Rehabilitation counseling services
13. School health services and school nurse services
14. Social work
15. Speech-language pathology
16. Transportation

Your child's IEP must include information about *when, where,* and *how frequently* your child will receive their services. Your Local Education Agency, or LEA (the school district), *is* responsible for funding and providing the related services your child needs. Your LEA will *not* fund medical treatment, ongoing health services, assistive technology for at-home use, or residential placement for non-education–related reasons.

WHO ARE THE SERVICE PROVIDERS?

Many adults might work with your child.

Here's an overview of who these adults are and the services they provide to children with disabilities in elementary school:

- **Case Manager:** Every child with an IEP has a case manager who is your point person for any questions, IEP-related or general ones about your child's learning. The case manager schedules meetings, manages paperwork, and communicates directly with you. Case managers reach out when your child is having a great day or when they need extra partnership from you. The case manager is usually the special education teacher, but in some situations, they may not be providing instruction.

- **Guidance Counselor:** These professionals support students' social and emotional well-being. They might provide individual counseling sessions to help students with anxiety, depression, friendship issues, or grief. Often, they facilitate small group counseling sessions or lunch bunches to help students with friendship and social skills. Guidance counselors lead whole-class lessons on anger management, decision making, friendship skills, relationship skills, and self-awareness.

- **Nurse:** School nurses promote health and well-being. They can administer medication to your child during the school day. (Most require the original bottle to be provided, as well as a note from the prescribing provider.) In addition to handling health emergencies and screenings, they assist students with chronic medical conditions, such as asthma, diabetes, or seizures.

- **Occupational Therapist, or OT:** OTs help students develop executive functioning, fine motor development, handwriting, self-regulation, or sensory processing skills. Often they provide students with adaptive equipment or technology, fine motor exercises, and sensory integration activities. OTs prepare students for academic success and independent living.

- **Paraeducator, or Para:** Paraeducators are credentialed individuals who work in schools under the supervision of licensed or certified professionals. These individuals support and assist students in various ways. Some paraeducators support students with academics, behavior, or language support to students learning English. They may also work one-on-one or lead small groups in general and special education classrooms. While paraeducators are not certified teachers, many have an associate's degree or certificate. They are essential members of the school community since they provide targeted student assistance. Sometimes, paraeducators go by other names, such as behavior technician, classroom aide, instructional assistant, nursing aide, one-to-one aide, paraprofessional, therapy assistant, or teacher assistant.

- **Physical Therapist, or PT:** PTs address physical limitations that hinder a child's participation in school activities. They address gross motor limitations and work with children to improve their balance, coordination, flexibility, or muscle strength. They may recommend assistive devices to help a child increase their independence at school.

- **Resource Teacher:** These teachers work with students who have special education needs. They provide individualized or small-group instruction, often in a resource room, but sometimes they support students by coming into their classroom to tailor lessons and materials to students' learning needs. Some resource teachers specialize in behavior support, providing social skills lessons, structured breaks, and specific support in a subject area that may trigger a child.

- **School Psychologist:** School psychologists support students' academic, behavioral, and social-emotional well-being. They assess and evaluate students, consult with teachers, collaborate to develop crisis intervention plans, and implement school-wide programs that prevent bullying and promote positive social-emotional learning and mental health awareness. Chapter 2 provides more details about school psychologists.

- **Social Worker:** School-based social workers support students' social-emotional well-being and overall development within a school setting. They collaborate with students, families, teachers, and other professionals to address various social, emotional, behavioral, and academic challenges that students may face. Social workers provide crisis intervention (with struggling students or families) and individual and group counseling.

- **Special Education Teacher:** Special educators ensure all students learn and flourish. They differentiate instruction by employing various strategies and methods for each child's learning style. They address learning disabilities and neurodivergence. These teachers can also help students develop emotional regulation strategies, foster executive functioning skills, and provide social skills instruction.

- **Speech-Language Pathologist, or SLP:** These professionals assess and treat students with communication disorders, including speech and language support. They might do articulation drills, language stimulation games, social skills training, work on self-advocacy skills, and provide reading comprehension strategies. They can also help improve students' conversational skills by teaching them to initiate conversations, actively listen, and practice turn-taking.

Sometimes **English as an Additional Language, or EAL,** teachers are on an IEP team since some kids are identified as English Language Learners and have a disability. EAL teachers instruct students learning English as an additional language by helping them develop their language skills and succeed academically.

UNDERSTANDING SPECIAL EDUCATION SUPPORT: IEPS VERSUS 504 PLANS

Schools create individualized educational programs (IEPs) and 504 Plans to support students with disabilities in elementary or secondary education.

The main difference is that an IEP is for students who require specialized instruction, while a 504 Plan is for students who don't need specialized instruction but still need accommodations to boost academic success and to make the learning environment more accessible. 504 Plans provide accommodations, but they do not include educational *goals*. Children who need an IEP and also have a medical condition that requires accommodations for academic success (or to make the learning environment safe, as in the case of a severe nut allergy) will have all of these needs addressed in the IEP. Your child will have either a 504 Plan or an IEP, not both.

The federal Individuals with Disabilities Education Act (IDEA) ensures that eligible children with disabilities can access special education and related services. As stated in Chapter 2, students must meet criteria in at least one of 13 categories of disabilities and require specialized instruction to have an IEP. As a result, an IEP is a more involved process and requires documentation of measurable growth.

A 504 Plan is part of a federal law called Section 504 of the Rehabilitation Act. This civil rights law protects individuals from discrimination due to their disability. A 504 Plan outlines specific accommodations students need to ensure they can fully participate in school.

Both IEPs and 504 Plans help students with disabilities succeed in school, but they're like two different apps on a smartphone.

IEPs are for students who need specialized instruction:

- Like a map, an IEP shows teachers how to help a student learn best.
- It could include smaller class sizes, one-on-one time, or unique materials.

- Each IEP contains specially designed instruction specific to a student's needs.

- The IEP requires documentation of measurable growth to track and monitor progress annually.

504 Plans are for students who need support and accommodations to remove barriers to learning:

- Like a wheelchair ramp, a 504 Plan doesn't change the classroom but lets a student access it easily.

- Accommodations are provided in the general education classroom so that a child can succeed in school by removing barriers for a student with a disability.

- In rare instances, 504 Plans may contain modifications or related services.

- Regular progress monitoring is not typically included in a 504 Plan since it focuses on accommodations rather than goals.

Both plans are updated annually to ensure the student receives the most effective support for their needs. The IEP team needs to review the student's IEP at least once a year. An IEP is a fluid document and can be updated more often if a student has met their goals or if their needs change before their annual review. A comprehensive review evaluates the child's need for continued services at three-year intervals and is sometimes called a *triennial*. Typically, a 504 Plan undergoes a yearly review and is reevaluated every three years or as necessary.

One of my goals in this book is to help parents understand the academic piece of their child's education—how a disability may impact academic progress and how to ensure that the assistance mandated by law provides the best possible help for an individual and unique child. Therefore, most chapters in the second part of this book will focus on IEPs, rather than 504 Plans. Even if your child has a 504 Plan, rather than an IEP, you'll find valuable information throughout the rest of this book.

For more information on 504 Plans, consult the resources at the back of the book.

Knowing the Distinction: 504 Plans versus IEPs

Determining whether your child needs a 504 Plan or an IEP is sometimes challenging. Conferring with your child's teacher or principal is a good first step.

However, to help you think through things beforehand, here are six scenarios of children needing a 504 Plan or an IEP.

Children Needing a 504 Plan in Elementary School

Because they are intended to ensure equal access to education, 504 Plans can be provided for any medical diagnosis that might compromise a child's education, not just learning disabilities and the like.

Scenario 1: ADHD and Sensory Processing Disorder

Caleb is a second grader who struggles to focus in class. He fidgets constantly, talks out of turn, and has difficulty following instructions. Caleb also has sensory processing disorder, which makes him sensitive to loud noises and bright lights.
Examples of 504 Plan accommodations:

- Preferential seating near the teacher or in a quiet classroom area
- Sensory breaks (for movement, for quiet, or for organization to get him ready to learn again)
- Access to fidget toys to help him focus
- Movement breaks to allow him to release energy
- Noise-canceling headphones to block out distracting noises
- Extra time to complete assignments

Scenario 2: Food Allergies

Juanita is a third-grade student with severe tree nut allergies. She must avoid tree nuts to prevent dangerous reactions.
Examples of 504 Plan accommodations:

- An emergency plan for allergic reactions in place at school and on field trips
- Tree-nut-free zones in the classroom to minimize exposure to allergens
- Education for teachers and classmates about food allergies and how to administer epinephrine
- Modified lunch arrangements to ensure Juanita has access to safe food options
- Permission to carry and use emergency medication

Scenario 3: Anxiety and Depression

Marielle is a fourth grader who struggles with anxiety and depression. She experiences frequent stomachaches, difficulty sleeping, and difficulty concentrating in school.

Examples of 504 Plan accommodations:

- Flexible schedule to allow for breaks and time to manage anxiety
- Quiet space to retreat when feeling overwhelmed
- A counselor or therapist who teaches relaxation techniques
- Reduced homework load or modified assignments
- Check-ins with a trusted adult to offer support.

Children Needing an IEP in Elementary School

Scenario 1: Autism Spectrum Disorder

Olivia is a kindergarten student with autism. She struggles with social interaction, communication, and repetitive behaviors.

Examples of IEP services:

- Specialized instruction in social skills and communication
- Visual schedules and routines to provide predictability and structure
- Positive reinforcement to promote success
- Occupational therapy to help with sensory processing issues
- Speech-language therapy to improve communication skills

Scenario 2: Intellectual Disability

Kristof is a first-grade student with an intellectual disability. He learns more slowly than his peers and needs additional support to access the general education curriculum.

Examples of IEP services:

- Modified curriculum with smaller learning steps and concrete examples
- Individualized instruction and support from a special education teacher
- Assistive technology tools to help with learning and communication

- Occupational therapy to improve fine motor skills
- Speech-language therapy to address any speech or language delays
- Paraeducator support in the classroom

Scenario 3: Visual Impairment

Thomas is a fifth grader with low vision. He needs specialized instruction and materials to access the learning environment.

Examples of IEP services:

- Enlarged print materials, audiobooks, text-to-speech software, and assistive technology tools to magnify text and images provide access to all aspects of his learning environment
- Orientation and mobility training to help navigate the school environment

These are just a few examples of children who may need 504 Plans or IEPs. It's important to remember that every child is unique, and their needs will vary. The specific services and supports are determined based on a comprehensive evaluation of the child's strengths, weaknesses, and learning style.

PULL-OUT VERSUS PUSH-IN INSTRUCTION

You'll hear the phrases "push-in" and "pull-out" support. These terms refer to where and how your child will receive specialized instruction and related services. When service providers *push into* a classroom, they're collaborating with the general education teacher in a way that allows them to support students' needs inside the general education classroom. A student who is *pulled out* of the general education classroom to work with the service provider in their classroom or office space will typically receive highly individualized instruction or services that are tailored to their needs.

I detested disruptions as a classroom teacher. I found it hard to focus on teaching when the phone was ringing, announcements were being made, and people were walking in and out of the classroom to get something or someone. If I had trouble focusing because of the distractions, I figured many of my students probably felt the same.

I solved the phone issue easily by asking my principal if I could take it off the hook during minilessons and independent work time. (We agreed someone would walk to my classroom with the message if something were urgent.) However, solving the revolving door of kids being pulled out of the classroom by the reading specialist, resource room teacher, social worker, speech therapist, and guidance counselor was tricky since pull-out support had always been the standard practice at my school.

I took this problem to my principal when I was a second-year teacher. I inquired about the possibility of some service providers pushing into my classroom to support my students during independent work times. He told me he couldn't change the structure of how things had been done, but permitted me to ask some of my colleagues if pushing in would be a possibility.

One of the reading specialists and the speech therapist agreed to push into my classroom to support some of my students. Over time, pushing in caused my students to miss less class time, which meant they stayed on track with their classwork.

As a general education teacher, I appreciated having service providers come to the classroom. This allowed them to listen to the same lesson the student heard me deliver, which was helpful so that the service providers knew what the child was working on. Much of the time, my colleagues were able and willing to bring whatever they needed to support the students on their caseload to my classroom so the child could stay in the classroom for independent work time. However, some service providers would stay for the minilesson and then pull their students out for part of their independent work time, allowing them to focus better in a smaller space. Once students had finished working independently, they returned to the classroom for a whole-class share and reflection time.

Some children do not want to be pulled out of the general education classroom to receive their services. For some of my former students, they feared being labeled as "different" or "stupid" by their peers. However, I've taught plenty of kids who preferred to be pulled out of their classroom to receive their services since they liked being one-on-one or in a small group with their peers, where it's usually a little quieter than the general education classroom.

I support a push-in model because it provides students with more opportunities to remain in the general education classroom. Pull-out support is justified if there's a legitimate rationale for pulling a child out of the classroom (for example, some kids work better in a classroom with fewer distractions or open up more when pulled out of the classroom).

It's important to ask *where* and *how* your child will be supported for their IEP goals. Pull-out support is often suggested since that might be the typical protocol at your child's school. Discuss options with the IEP team if you're hesitant about disrupting your child's schedule or want them to be in the least restrictive environment, which is the general education classroom for most children.

THE DIFFERENCES BETWEEN ACCOMMODATIONS AND MODIFICATIONS

You'll likely hear the buzzwords *accommodation* and *modification* during an IEP meeting. It's essential to understand the difference between the words since they serve very different purposes. An accommodation is *how* the student accesses their learning and the school environment. A modification is *what* the student is taught or expected to learn.

> Accommodations specify *how* students get what they need to learn; modifications specify *what* they learn.

Modifications are controversial since they can vastly alter how much a child learns (Hehir, 2017). Some modifications alter expectations. For instance, in English Language Arts, a reading modification could be providing a child with a text written at their reading level rather than their grade level. A writing modification could be a reduction in the number of paragraphs a child needs in an essay. In word study, they may be taught and tested on fewer words. Modifications are often necessary if a child is working far below grade level. However, the bottom line is that *the more modifications there are, the less exposure the child has to the curriculum.* Over time, this can profoundly impact how much a child learns, which can potentially impact them on standardized college entrance exams like the ACT and SAT or on showcasing their mastery on state-level exams based on what is taught in high school, which could thereby impact their ability to obtain their high school diploma. While high school graduation is a long way off for your child, it's prudent to follow the advice of Tom Hehir, EdD, to start with accommodations and follow with modifications only when necessary.

Examples of Accommodations and Modifications

Accommodations help students complete the same tasks as their peers but with some changes in time, format, setting, or presentation. Accommodations aim to ensure students have an equal chance to learn and demonstrate their knowledge and abilities.

- Provide guided notes
- Use a calculator on math assignments
- Have someone read a test aloud (except when reading comprehension is being assessed)
- Preferential seating (for example, away from distractions like doors, speakers, and windows; near the teacher)
- Pair visuals alongside spoken information
- Time warnings and increased transition time
- Advance notice of drills (such as fire, intruder)
- Provide audio and video recordings
- Use of fidget toys
- Use clear, concise instructions or directions
- Provide extra time for the student to process information; teach peers how to give the student extra wait time.
- Provide sensory breaks
- Extend allotted time on assessments (such as time and a half, double time)
- Use alarms on a device for reminders
- Provide visual routines and schedules

Modifications change parts of an assignment or adjust what students are supposed to learn based on their abilities. Students with modifications don't have to learn all the same things as their peers since they have different learning goals.

- Reword test questions with straightforward language
- Learn different material (continue working on a skill that hasn't been mastered while classmates move on to a different unit, for example)
- Provide books with the same content but at a simpler reading level
- Limit multiple-choice answers to three responses
- Permit calculators on math tests
- Receive alternate assignments or projects
- Complete less or different homework than classmates
- Allow oral testing
- Give a word bank with choices to assist with answering test questions
- Receive adult assistance on assignments
- Modify deadlines
- Receive tests based on different standards than classmates
- Test spelling separately from written content
- Answer different test questions than peers
- Provide a pass/no pass option

In the fifth grade, Bao transitioned to an urban public school when her family moved from a different part of their state. Her mom, Liên, requested a meeting with her case manager the week before school began to ensure they were on the same page with Bao's IEP.

Her case manager brought Bao's IEP to the table with sticky notes peeking out of many pages. She noticed Liên looking at the sticky notes when she quickly said, "I tabbed all of the parts I want to discuss with you today."

"As a fellow sticky note user and Bao's mom, I appreciate your reviewing the IEP thoroughly before our meeting."

She shrugged as if to say, "That's what I do."

Once they arrived at the pages containing the supports that would be provided to Bao, she looked at Liên and said, "Most of this is just good teaching, but I want to review some of them with you to make sure I'm clear."

"I agree. Unfortunately, many of these accommodations were the outgrowth of things that weren't happening in Bao's old school."

They went through the list item by item. As Bao's teacher read through them, she kept saying, "Well, this is just good teaching."

The repetition of "These things are just good teaching" increased Liên's confidence in Bao's new teacher. She got it! She repeatedly communicated that to Liên and told her Bao was in for a good year. Her case manager was perplexed by the inclusion of many items listed on the specially designed instruction pages of her IEP.

Yet, at the annual meeting, most of those items stayed on the IEP, and several new accommodations were added once Bao's case manager got to know her better. Why? Liên thinks the case manager knew others would need a roadmap when working with Bao as she transitioned to middle school.

EVERYTHING DOESN'T ALWAYS GO WELL

Sometimes the school and the parent do not see eye to eye during the IEP process. You can and should speak up if something doesn't feel right or if you have a major disagreement and the school won't provide something you think your child needs.

After an IEP meeting, your child's case manager will issue a Notice of Recommended Educational Placement/Prior Written Notice, or NOREP/ PWN. You have 10 days (some states use calendar days, while others use school days) to respond to the NOREP/PWN to approve or disapprove the recommendations.

TIP

Caution: Your child's school can proceed with the recommendations in the NOREP/PWN if you do not sign and return it by the specified date.

If you disagree with the changes suggested in NOREP/PWN, requesting a due process hearing or mediation within 10 days is crucial to prevent the changes from happening without your consent. You can inform the school about your disagreement by filling out the "do not approve" section of the NOREP/PWN and asking for mediation or due process. Telling the school you disapprove will prevent the changes and protect your rights.

You have three courses of action when this occurs:

- **Informal Meeting:** An informal meeting aims to facilitate open dialogue and problem solving between parents and the IEP team when they disagree. This meeting provides a platform to clarify concerns, understand each other's perspectives, explore alternative solutions, and maintain a positive working relationship. While the outcome is not legally binding, this collaborative approach helps address disagreements more efficiently, avoiding the need for formal dispute resolution processes that can be stressful and costly. It's important to note that the result of an informal meeting is not legally binding. Parents can still pursue other dispute resolution avenues, such as mediation or due process, if an agreement is not reached.

- **Mediation:** Mediation seeks to facilitate a collaborative and constructive discussion to reach a mutually agreeable solution when a parent disagrees with the IEP team. Mediation can be valuable for resolving IEP disagreements because it facilitates open communication, explores solutions, avoids costly expenses, promotes positive relationships, and protects the child's right to a FAPE. A neutral mediator guides the conversation between the parent and the school district. Mediation aims to maintain or improve the working relationship between parents and the IEP team. The outcome of mediation is not final. The parents and the IEP team must agree to any solutions proposed during mediation. If they can't reach an agreement, parents can still consider other options like a due process hearing or filing a complaint with an education agency.

- **Due Process:** Parents who believe the services offered or provided by the school are unsuitable, or who disagree with the proposed placement or the school's decision that their child is not eligible for services, can ask for a due process hearing. Due process is a formal, private legal proceeding. It involves a hearing officer who listens to both sides, reviews evidence, and makes an impartial decision. This process ensures a fair and impartial resolution, protects the child's and parents' rights, allows for the presentation of evidence and expert opinions, and results in a final and binding decision. If either party disagrees with the due process decision, they can file a civil lawsuit within 90 days.

In addition, you can file a written state complaint if you believe a school has violated a requirement of the Individuals with Disabilities Education Act (IDEA).

The complaint should be written directly to the State Education Agency (SEA), describing the violation, and must be signed. The school system can respond to the complaint and propose a resolution. The SEA typically has 60 calendar days to resolve the complaint and provide a written decision addressing each allegation and explaining the reasons for the decision. If the SEA finds that the school failed to provide appropriate services, it must take corrective action, such as compensatory services or reimbursement, to meet the child's needs. (Compensatory services are provided to students with disabilities when they miss out on learning because their school didn't provide the services delineated in their IEP.)

The Center for Appropriate Dispute Resolution in Special Education (CADRE) has a comparison chart, "Quick Guide to Special Education Dispute Resolution Processes for Parents of Children & Youth (Ages 3–21)," to help parents decide when to use each type of dispute resolution with the child's school. Not only does this chart explain process distinctions, time frames, and financial costs, but it also illustrates the impact each type of dispute resolution has on relationships with the school. (See Resources.)

Anti-Discrimination and Access Protection via Section 504

Section 504 of the Rehabilitation Act also safeguards students with disabilities against discrimination. Section 504 provides additional options for addressing any issues. You can file a complaint with the Office for Civil Rights, or OCR, part of the U.S. Department of Education. (The complaint filing process might change due to the Department of Education changes initiated in 2025).

You must file an OCR complaint within 180 days of the school's violation. An OCR complaint can initiate an investigation into the school's actions.

Check the Resources to learn more about OCR complaints.

As an educator and parent, I know that disagreement and conflict are an inevitable part of ongoing relationships. It's essential to start with the least contentious option since that preserves relationships and is most likely to benefit your child's outcomes in the classroom more quickly. My belief is rooted in the notion that schools strive to provide the best for all children.

There is a time and place for mediation, due process, and written complaints to state agencies. These are proven ways to help you get what your child deserves if the school will not willingly provide accommodations, modifications, or related services you believe your child needs to thrive. However, filing a SEA complaint can be perceived as adversarial and may potentially escalate or intensify a situation, much like due process.

Most school district employees don't wake up on a Tuesday and say, "I want to make life hard for this family." Rather, most LEAs want to get you what your child needs. However, if your LEA is being adversarial or looking at your child with dollar signs (that is, how much money your child's services and supports will cost them), you are within your rights to escalate your concerns to a higher entity.

> **TIP** Remember, resolutions take time. Finding an easy and efficient solution to school-related problems is often unlikely. If straightforward fixes were available, the school and the parents would have likely discovered them already. Complicated issues tend to require more time and effort to address. For instance, a complaint filed through the State Education Agency typically takes 60 days to process, which accounts for approximately one-third of your child's school year. Due process usually takes around 45 days. However, it often extends to 90 days, effectively taking up half of the school year. If the situation escalates to litigation, it can take one to two years to resolve. Meanwhile, your child's needs also have to be met during this extended period.

Getting Assistance

Several national organizations can support you with legal assistance or advocates:

- Council of Parents and Attorneys, or COPAA, is an organization that helps parents find advocates and attorneys to represent them in special education situations. It can be considered a national clearinghouse for advocates and attorneys since it has a code of ethics for its members.

- There are 57 Protection and Advocacy, or P&A, agencies in the United States which operate under the auspices of the National Disability Rights Network. P&As provide direct advocacy by working with parents to attend IEP meetings, due process hearings, or other informal negotiations. Attorneys from a P&A can go to state or federal court to advocate for a student's rights. Because P&As address barriers a person has *because* of their disability, they are selective about the cases they take. They have limited staffing and funding, so they only take on cases that have legal merit and fit their current focus areas. (You can find your P&A's focus areas by searching for their goals and objectives. An example of the Minnesota Disability Law Center's Statement of Goals and Priorities can be found in the Resources.)

- The Advocacy Institute is a nonprofit organization that provides many resources to help you advocate for your child. A particularly noteworthy feature on their website is the IDEA State Complaint Resource Center, a hub for information, resources, and support in utilizing the IDEA Written State Complaint process. It contains details on the complaint process, including podcasts, webinars, and video presentations. You can explore state-specific data on filed complaints, find direct links to written complaint procedures for each state, and browse a topic-based bank of state complaints.

PRIVATE SCHOOL VERSUS PUBLIC SCHOOL

Carlos attended private school through third grade. His parents, Bryan and Liz, opted to send him there instead of public school because the class sizes were small. They had heard, from a parent who had a child with a disability, that the school would be flexible with them when Carlos had to miss school for things like occupational and physical therapy.

And they were. But there was still a problem.

Carlos didn't have regular access to school-based support services. For instance, a reading specialist (not employed by the school but rather by a local agency) agreed to see Carlos weekly. While that seemed helpful, Carlos missed many sessions with her since she only came to Carlos's school on Mondays. During a typical fall, a couple of Mondays are off for national holidays, plus a fall break. This meant Carlos didn't receive pull-out reading instruction multiple times that fall.

You might think Carlos's services would be available on another weekday. Unfortunately, that wasn't the case since the agency's reading specialist was scheduled in other schools each weekday. Since Carlos was in private school, his school had no IEP to follow. Therefore, they were not mandated by law to provide Carlos with learning support.

Plus, a limited amount of money is available to fund outside professionals coming into the school to provide learning support services to private school students. If his parents wanted to have Carlos supported, they'd have to seek external tutoring for him at their expense—or send him to public school.

While some private schools exist to educate students who learn and think differently, most do not provide the level of support public schools provide. Nonpublic schools are not required by law to provide special education services.

The Department of Education provided updated guidance, "Questions and Answers on Serving Children with Disabilities Placed by Their Parents in Private Schools," in 2022. This "Q&A document guides parents concerning IDEA requirements that apply to disabled children who attend private schools." While private school students have some rights (such as the right to be evaluated for a disability), the bottom line is that many private schools do not provide the level of support many kids with disabilities need.

Some private schools offer learning support centers, teachers with extra training for students with learning disabilities, and other services to help children with learning and thinking differences progress. It's important to have candid conversations with the admissions officer to determine what the school can offer for your child. Some potential questions are:

- Will the school create a learning plan for my child? Tell me about that process. How do you monitor progress?
- What kinds of training do your teachers have to support students with learning and thinking differences similar to my child?
- Will my child be supported with a push-in model, a pull-out model, or both?
- What kinds of accommodations do you provide for children like mine?
- Do you have a guidance counselor or school psychologist who supports mental health?
- Are there extra fees for counseling, mobility services, speech-language therapy?

It's important to note that the rare private schools for children who think and learn differently often have exorbitant price tags. It's worth looking into those schools if you can afford the tuition or will qualify for financial aid.

Finally, tap into your network of other friends, family, support groups, and even online groups to get the scoop on what local schools can offer your child. Gather your information from several sources to make a decision that's in your child's best interest if you're considering sending them to a private school.

With every passing year Carlos was in private school, parents Bryan and Liz heard whisperings about parents who pulled their child from private school to attend public school since the private school could not meet their needs with a tiny faculty and little external support for things like counseling and reading specialists. These students needed services during the school day to help them with their learning disabilities. They eventually became part of this small group of parents who pulled their children out of private school to get an IEP in public school, which would entitle them to the appropriate amount of services for their disabilities.

Once they realized private school wouldn't be in Carlos's best interest long-term and realized they couldn't afford to send him to a specialized school for children with learning disabilities in their city, they began looking into public school districts where people in their parent network flocked instead of to private school. Many public elementary schools are known for providing above-average support to students with learning disabilities. By talking to people in their parent and professional networks, Bryan and Liz were able to get nonpublicized information to help them find an elementary school that would be a better fit for their son.

CHARTER SCHOOLS

Charter schools are public schools that allow families to choose an educational option that best fits their child's needs. Attending is free since charter schools are publicly funded. They're open to all, but a lottery system is usually in place, so the admissions process is fair and unbiased. These innovative public schools are led by administrators who can experiment with new approaches. (Charters often have more flexibility within the state but are still restricted by federal regulations.) To maintain the flexibility and independence granted to it, the charter school must adhere to the accountability requirements specified in its charter agreement.

Many parents consider charter schools since they feel they aren't getting something their child needs at their local public school. I debated sharing my thoughts on charter schools in general since I taught fourth grade at a well-respected public charter school in Rhode Island. Several of my students had IEPs and received high-quality push-in and pull-out support for counseling, math, OT, reading, speech, and writing. The school community was nurturing and welcoming to all students, regardless of their income level, knowledge of English, or disability.

However, over the years, I've heard plenty of stories about children being pushed out of charter schools because they have higher support needs.

There are phenomenal charter schools out there, but there are also charter schools that don't want to serve "those kids." To keep a charter open, they have to meet certain thresholds. They may not be able to do this if they serve many students with higher support needs. One of the things they'll do is say something like, *we don't think we can serve your child here*. It's a real strategy, a real thing, a real practice that happens. While charter schools shouldn't be allowed to cherry-pick their kids, some do.

There are different kinds of charter schools. A single-operating charter school manages itself. Then there are nonprofit and for-profit organizations and networks that run charter schools. Knowing the type of charter you're considering for your child is essential before you apply. You can research the school online and speak with its administrators. I strongly suggest you talk to other parents of children with disabilities whose kids go to a charter school you're interested in to get a sense of whether or not the school would be able to meet your child's support needs.

You can find resources at the back of the book to help you learn about charter schools.

FROM IEP TO IMPLEMENTATION

You now have the lay of the IEP land! (It's a lot, I know.) I hope this chapter has helped you understand the landscape so you can make well-informed decisions on your child's behalf.

Next, we'll continue navigating the education maze by looking at where your child gets services, how your LEA classifies them, and what accommodations and modifications they'll receive.

Tip for Cultivating Joy: Bring on the joy by creating playlists for relaxation, a pick-me-up, to boost your spirits, or to enjoy with your child. Cue the needed playlist in the background, sing along, or dance to whatever music makes you joyful.

Self-Care Tip: Journaling helps you process your thoughts, problem-solve, reflect on what's happening with your child, and can help with stress reduction. You don't need anything fancy to get started! A simple spiral notebook and a writing utensil or a new document on your device/computer is all you need to start writing. While you don't have to write at a specific time, it helps to schedule a regular time to do some writing. Start by blocking off 10 minutes to write. You'll find links to journaling resources at the back of the book.

4

Know What Your Child Will Receive

"Special education is a service or support students receive, but it isn't who they are." A child's potential shouldn't be defined or limited based on being a "special education student." Children receiving special education services have unique learning or higher support needs. An aspect of one's education should not define one's identity. A more appropriate term would be *accessible education,* emphasizing the goal of making education accessible to all students. A shift in language would signal that education is accessible to all learners.

When we stop categorizing students as "special education students," we encourage a more inclusive approach, where all students are seen as individuals with diverse strengths and abilities. Children with disabilities should be recognized for their full range of talents and potential rather than being defined solely by their need for educational support.

As a literacy consultant, I cringe when I meet with educators who refer to their students as "IEP kids" or "my special ed kids." Rather than calling these folks out, I attempt to call them in *privately,* using a technique Loretta J. Ross, a human rights educator, explains:

> Calling in is a technique that does allow all parties to move forward. It's a concept created by human-rights practitioners to challenge the toxicity of call-out culture. Calling in is speaking up without tearing down. A call-in can happen publicly or privately, but its key feature is that it's done with

love. Instead of shaming someone who's made a mistake, we can patiently ask questions to explore what was going on and why the speaker chose their harmful language.

Often, teachers don't realize how their language minimizes their students. I've been known to pause a one-on-one conversation or talk to the teacher privately in a debrief. I might begin with "How would you say _____ if one of your students or their parents were with us in the room?" or "I think it might be helpful to reframe _____. Let's go back for a moment and talk about some inclusive language I use to talk about students with different learning needs." These openings lead to a conversation that helps teachers speak more inclusively and respectfully about their students.

However, as parents, we need to remember that it starts with us. Many of us talk about our children in a way that doesn't see the whole person. Saying things like "I have a special needs kid" defines our children by only part of who they are—their disability.

Tiffany Yu includes some excellent prompting questions for *calling in* people in The Anti-Ableist Manifesto. You can try some of the following whenever necessary:

- What do you mean when you say that?
- What are the assumptions you're making when you use those words?
- What preconceived notions do you have about disability?
- Have you listened to a disabled person about to learn more what their reality/situation is like?

Maritza, age nine, has a **specific learning disability in mathematics** and received an initial IEP during the first marking period of fourth grade. Her IEP team proposed to have Maritza pulled out of the general education classroom for daily reteaching of math concepts for 30 minutes. Maritza would receive special education services, provided by special education personnel (that is, a special educator and paraeducators), for 20% or less of the school day.

The IEP team shared the following specially designed instruction, which included the following:

- Receive small group, direct instruction in math.
- Provide enlarged graph paper when completing math calculations to aid in organizing columns and rows.

- Receive visual aids (such as math keyword charts, multiplication tables, facts) to reduce demands when solving math problems.
- Chunk of assignments so the simplest task is presented first to ensure success.

Maritza's parents felt 30 minutes per day was not enough to address Maritza's math struggles since she was performing far below grade level. During Maritza's IEP adoption meeting, they asked if Maritza could get more time with a special educator. The IEP team insisted that 30 minutes in the learning support classroom would be enough time to reteach concepts and catch her up. Plus, being pulled out for only 30 minutes of a 90-minute math block meant that Maritza would be in the least restrictive environment.

Maritza's parents remained skeptical but didn't want to push too hard. The case manager suggested that Maritza begin with the 30-minute daily reteach time and they reconvene for an informal meeting in three months to assess how Maritza was progressing with her math application goal. Not wanting to be too adversarial, Maritza's parents agreed to the amount of special education services the IEP team suggested.

LEARNING IN THE LEAST RESTRICTIVE ENVIRONMENT

One key principle of the Individuals with Disabilities Education Act (IDEA) is that children should be educated in the least restrictive environment, or LRE. This means children who receive special education should be alongside their peers in the general education classroom as much as possible.

These are the general LRE requirements from IDEA:

(2) Each public agency must ensure that—
   (i) To the maximum extent appropriate, children with disabilities, including children in public or private institutions or other care facilities, are educated with children who are nondisabled; and
   (ii) Special classes, separate schooling, or other removal of children with disabilities from the regular educational environment occurs only if the nature or severity of the disability is such that education in regular classes with the use of supplementary aids and services cannot be achieved satisfactorily.

(Sec. 300.114 LRE requirements, *https://sites.ed.gov/ idea/regs/b/b/300.114*)

The general education setting is typically considered the standard LRE. IDEA makes it clear that the general education classroom and curriculum are where students with disabilities should be unless they're unable to meet their goals.

You can think of LRE as a spectrum since a range of educational placements is available for students with disabilities. The most appropriate setting should be determined based on each student's needs. A student's LRE can vary throughout the school day depending on their instructional content and settings, as certain students with specific learning needs may require different environments to best support their education.

Parents should be involved in all conversations concerning their child's educational placement since *every child has the right to be included*. When placing a child, the IEP team, which you are part of, must prioritize the child's inclusion in various experiences alongside nondisabled children, including academics and extracurricular activities.

The National Center for Education Statistics tracks the number of students, ages 3–21, who receive IDEA services in the United States. The number increased from 6.4 million during the 2010–11 school year to 7.3 million in the 2021–22 school year. The table below provides a look at the daily percentage of support students receive in a typical day.

Percentage of School Day That Students Received Support

Educational Environment	2010–11	2021–22
Less than 40% of the school day spent in general education (aka: full-time support)	14%	13%
41–79% of the school day spent in general education (aka: supplemental support)	20%	16%
80% or more of the school day spent in general education	61%	67%

Source: https://nces.ed.gov/programs/coe/indicator/cgg/students-with-disabilities

In a decade, the percentage of students who spent 80% or more of their time in general education classes, considered the least restrictive environment, increased from 61 to 67%.

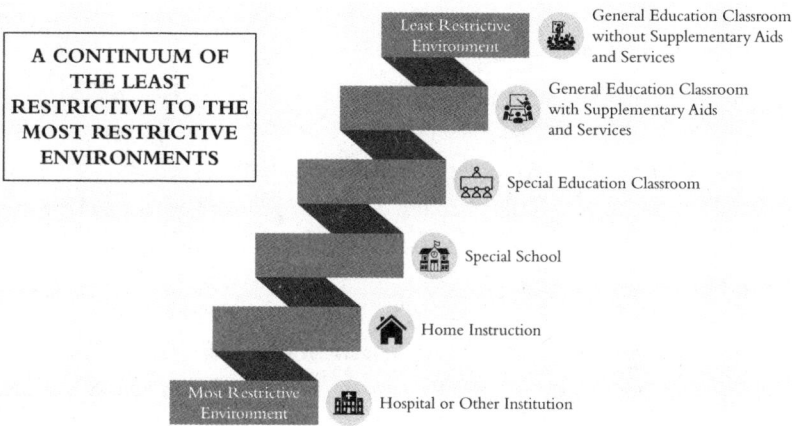

A CONTINUUM OF THE LEAST RESTRICTIVE TO THE MOST RESTRICTIVE ENVIRONMENTS

Least Restrictive Environment

General Education Classroom without Supplementary Aids and Services

General Education Classroom with Supplementary Aids and Services

Special Education Classroom

Special School

Home Instruction

Most Restrictive Environment

Hospital or Other Institution

A Closer Look at Each Setting

What do the environments shown in the box look like for children being educated there?

General Education Classroom with Supplementary Aids and Services

In this setting, the general education teacher provides instruction with accommodations and modifications for the student. Instruction is supported with specialized materials, equipment, or methods.

Students may receive instruction in the general education classroom with support from a special education teacher. The general education teacher provides most, if not all, instruction with accommodations or modifications as needed. The special education teacher provides consultation, collaboration, and individualized/small-group instruction based on the student's needs. In some schools, students may be in a class co-taught by two certified educators.

Special Education Classroom

Part-Time

A student may receive supplemental instruction in a special education classroom for part of the school day. Some of the child's instruction occurs in the general education classroom with accommodations or modifications by the general education teacher. Special education services may include individual/small-group instruction in a separate room (resource room or learning support). For example, a student might be pulled out of the classroom to work with a reading specialist or receive full-replacement mathematics instruction in a smaller environment, while the rest of their day is spent in the general education classroom.

Full-Time

Most instruction occurs in the special education classroom. General education teachers, including those in nonacademic periods (like art or physical education), consult the special education teacher for effective instruction/support. Special education services may include specialized instruction in a self-contained classroom for students with similar needs, using specialized teaching strategies, assistive technologies, adaptive materials, and individualized support services.

Various types of support are available to students with disabilities, and an Individualized Education Program (IEP) Team can determine which is best based on the student's specific needs.

- Autistic support
- Blind and visually impaired support
- Emotional support
- Deaf and hearing-impaired support
- Learning support
- Life skills support
- Multiple disabilities support
- Physical support
- Speech and language support

An IEP team may decide that more than one type of support for a student's disabilities is necessary. This decision ensures that the student's unique, specific needs are adequately met so that they receive the necessary support for their educational journey.

Special School

Students receive their education in a separate school catering to students with similar disability-related needs. The educational setting is specifically designed, staffed, and equipped to provide appropriate care and education for these students. Ideally, these schools are close to a student's home so they can return home at night. There are residential options as well.

Home Instruction

Instruction conducted in the home means teachers provide individualized instruction according to the student's schedule and collaborate with general and special education teachers to plan and deliver instruction. It is an extremely restrictive alternative placement since the child has no exposure to general education settings. This placement is *not* homeschooling since the school district, not the parent, instructs the child.

Hospital or Other Institution

Hospital

Students receive instruction in a hospital for most of the school day. Hospitalized students have physical or mental health challenges requiring an extended stay. Education professionals in the hospital provide individualized instruction based on the student's schedule and collaborate with general and special education teachers to plan and deliver instruction.

Other Institution

Students receive instruction in a residential facility. Some students with significant physical or mental health challenges require the specialized services offered in these facilities.

Maritza's parents attended the three-month follow-up meeting to discuss Maritza's progress toward her math application goal. Maritza's case manager shared some areas of strength regarding Maritza's mastery of addition and subtraction facts with automaticity. However, Maritza was not developing an automaticity with multiplication or division, nor were word problems solved accurately if they involved more than one step. Maritza was given probes, short assessments used to check her understanding of math concepts, at a second-grade level every other week. The goal was for her to score 85% or higher on two out of three consecutive probes. While Maritza did well on some probes, most of her scores fell short of the 85% threshold. Nothing was consecutive. Plus, Maritza received grades in the 60s on math tests given by her general education teacher.

"What else can you do to help Maritza so she doesn't fall further behind?" Maritza's parents asked with concern.

The IEP team added accommodations:

- Provide opportunities to talk through the strategies or problem-solving steps Maritza is using with a teacher for the current math concept she is working on
- Have word problems read aloud
- Give her extra workspace on the paper to solve math problems
- Provide extended time on assessments

Maritza's mom had not inquired about the availability of co-taught math classes with two teachers. Although they had asked about having a paraeducator support Maritza in the classroom, the school responded that there were no staff members available for additional assistance, which led to frustration about the situation.

Maritza was set to receive 30 minutes of small group support to help her grasp grade-level concepts from the general education classroom, but her mother was concerned it wasn't enough. Her mom planned to evaluate Maritza's progress at the end of the school year and hoped the additional accommodations would be beneficial. Although it was suggested that they could request more frequent IEP meetings, Maritza's mother is reluctant to do so, believing the teachers know what is best. She indicated that they would consider calling a meeting if issues arise.

"They're still going to give Maritza 30 minutes of small group support to reteach the grade-level concepts she is learning in the general education classroom. But, honestly, I don't think that's enough," she told me forlornly. Then she added, "I guess we'll see how things are going once the school year finishes. Maybe she'll progress with these extra accommodations."

"Did you know you can call more frequent IEP meetings? As a parent, this is your right," I offered.

"I don't want to be too demanding. They're the teachers; they know best."

"True," I said gently. "But you know your child best. You won't offend anyone if you call for a meeting sooner."

"We'll see. If things become more of a problem, we'll call one."

PROMOTING THE OPTIMAL LEARNING ENVIRONMENT

It's important to note that LRE doesn't refer to a specific place or location. Instead, it involves deciding on the services and support a student needs to succeed and determining how and where those services can be provided effectively.

Knowing how many minutes your child will spend in and outside the general education setting is essential. The options for *where* a student is placed can change. Your child might get some services in one place and others in another. In addition, placements can change over time depending on the student's progress or needs. See the box below for questions to ask about your child's placement.

Questions to Ask about Your Child's Placement

- What are my child's needs?
- How can my child's needs be met in the least restrictive ways?
- Can my child receive a satisfactory education in the general education classroom to meet their needs?
- If so, what supplementary aids and supports will be put in place for my child to make progress on their IEP goals?
- If not, what percentage of the time will they be in the general education setting?

The IEP team discusses the specific instructional program and supports the student's needs based on their current abilities and areas of strength and weakness. These services and supports aim to help the student achieve their academic or functional goals, participate in the general education curriculum, and engage in extracurricular and nonacademic activities alongside their peers, both with and without disabilities. In cases where a child's disability hampers them from making satisfactory progress in the LRE, even with additional support, they might be placed in a more restrictive setting to ensure they receive an appropriate education. The general education classroom might not be the least restrictive option for some students. Moving to a more restrictive environment will happen only as necessary; returning to a less restrictive environment happens more quickly.

Many schools will assign a paraeducator to work with the student as a one-on-one aide or to provide instructional assistance, which has been described as "the most restrictive option within a general education classroom—an example of 'excluding practices in an inclusive setting'" (Jung, Frey, Fisher, and Kroener, 2019). Rather than assigning a para to a disabled student who learns in an inclusive general education classroom, the authors of *Your Students, My Students, Our Students: Rethinking Equitable and Inclusive Classrooms* assert that having a paraeducator work with an entire class is a better way. This makes the para's presence less likely to limit the disabled student's social opportunities. So while they provide intermittent support to students with IEPs, paraeducators can benefit all students by helping a teacher reteach concepts to small groups, facilitate station teaching (a co-teaching model where students rotate through various learning stations), or provide functional support.

It was almost the bitter end of fourth grade, and Maritza's parents were more worried than before. Despite their spending 10 minutes a day working with Maritza to memorize basic facts, she still wasn't making reasonable progress. She was not showing mastery on in-class tests and the probes. Plus, Maritza was engaging in negative self-talk, calling herself the "stupidest kid in the class" and saying she was "bad at math." Her parents reported that she grew agitated whenever they wanted to go over incorrect test problems with her at home.

At the IEP team meeting they requested, Maritza's dad said, "This isn't working. I'm worried about Maritza's self-esteem. She shouldn't come home and feel she's slower than the rest of her peers because she has a learning disability that makes math hard. She needs more help."

After a beat, Maritza's mom added, "We understand the law says that she should spend most of her day in the general education classroom, but she's not getting ahead. It feels like she's falling further behind. Can we talk about getting her more support from her classroom during the math block?"

After several minutes of back and forth, the IEP team decided that at the beginning of fifth grade, Maritza would be pulled out of her classroom for the full math block (90 minutes/day) to receive all math instruction from a special educator in a learning support classroom, which would mean more time in a special education setting. In addition, the IEP team suggested Maritza meet with the school's guidance counselor for the first marking period of the next school year to address some of the negative feelings she had developed as a result of her difficulties with math. While this kind of part-time learning support would mean less time with nondisabled peers, Maritza's IEP team concluded that part-time learning support could benefit her more in the long run.

Maritza's mom said, "I'm glad we didn't wait until her annual IEP renewal meeting. I think starting the next school year with more support will help Maritza. We'll see what happens at her annual IEP meeting this fall."

A child's educational placement is reviewed at least once a year, where their Individualized Education Program (IEP) and their current abilities, strengths, and areas where support is needed will be considered.

BENEFITS OF CO-TEACHING

I began my teaching career in the New York City Public Schools. I had the privilege of observing in collaborative team teaching, or CTT, classrooms several times. I remember a primary classroom where the general and special educators collaborated seamlessly to reach their students. The class was evenly split between children who had identified disabilities and nondisabled students. The special educator wasn't just delivering specially designed instruction. **Both** teachers took ownership of all the students by team teaching, having station rotations, and assisting with behavioral needs while each other taught. Watching the synergy in their classroom was beautiful since their students regarded them as equals. Both teachers were every child's teacher.

All children have the right to access the grade-level curriculum and to be educated alongside their same-age, typically developing peers to the greatest extent possible. One way to make this happen is to ask if your child's school offers co-taught classes (sometimes called *collaborative team teaching* or *integrated co-teaching*). Two certified teachers teach these classes: a general educator and a special educator. Both teachers work together to adapt or modify the content. Delivering specialized instruction helps all their students access the same curriculum as their grade-level peers.

Marilyn Friend delineated six models for co-teaching in her book on educational collaboration skills. Here are the basics to know so you can ask questions about the co-teaching models your child's school uses before agreeing to place them in a co-taught class:

- **Alternative (Differentiated) Teaching**: one teacher instructs most students, while the other focuses on a small group with specific needs. One teacher handles the large group, while the other targets a smaller group for various purposes such as enrichment, remediation, assessment, preteaching, or alternative teaching methods.

- **One Teaches, One Assists:** one teacher directly instructs students while the other provides individual assistance and support. The primary teacher leads the instruction while the assisting teacher monitors student work, addresses behavior issues, answers student questions, distributes materials, and seeks clarification from the lead teacher when necessary.

- **One Teaches, One Observes:** one teacher provides direct instruction to students while the other focuses on observing students' learning. The primary teacher delivers the instruction, while the observing teacher gathers specific information on students' academic, behavioral, and social skills within the classroom. Roles can be switched based on the topic or interests of the teachers, but this strategy is intended for occasional use.

- **Parallel Teaching:** co-teachers divide the class in half and instruct each group on the identical material simultaneously, without rotating the groups. This approach allows for a lower student-teacher ratio and increased student participation.

- **Station Teaching:** co-teachers divide the class into small groups, and each teacher provides instruction at a separate station, covering specific parts of the content. The activities at each station are designed to function independently and take approximately the same amount of time, allowing student groups to rotate between stations. This approach reduces the student-teacher ratio and enables monitoring of students' progress.

- **Team Teaching:** both teachers actively instruct students simultaneously. They share the responsibilities of leading instruction and may be at the front of the classroom, each with their distinct roles in the lesson. This approach promotes teacher collaboration and brings energy to the classroom, which benefits student engagement.

Questions to Ask About Co-Teaching

- Which co-teaching models do you use?
- Do you combine different types?
- How do you decide which to use?

Models *can and should* vary throughout the school day. Knowing the different models, you can ask questions to help you understand how the special education teacher will deliver your child's specially designed instruction in a co-taught class.

INFORMED PLACEMENT DECISIONS

As children, we learn about *wh-* questions. To better understand your child's IEP, it's important to get the answers to the following *wh-* questions:

- Who will deliver instruction to my child? Who will they be educated with?
- What does my child need to be successful with the general education curriculum?
- What kind of services will my child receive?
- What is the rationale for removing my child from the general education setting to receive intervention?
- When will my child receive the services they're entitled to in their IEP? How much time will they receive specialized instruction to help them meet their IEP goals?
- Where will my child be educated in the school, and is that the most natural setting for them to receive their services?
- What kind of training does the paraeducator have (if they provide part of my child's services)?

- Why have these people, services, time frames, and locations been selected for my child? What qualifications make these people uniquely positioned to provide this instruction?

Regardless of your child's disability, it's important to get the answers to these questions because schools must support students by thoughtfully planning for their needs. Elementary schools that want to provide children with disabilities with a strong foundation to succeed and belong in school and beyond will work with you to create an inclusive environment for your child.

FROM SPECIAL TO INCLUSIVE: REFRAMING EDUCATION

Special education, the term commonly used in the United States, is inherently problematic as it "others" students with disabilities. (Othering is treating people or a group as intrinsically different.) As noted at the beginning of this chapter, a more appropriate term would be *accessible education*.

An inclusion philosophy drives an effective school system. Creating a culture of equity and inclusion requires sharing research about its effectiveness, disrupting beliefs about disability, and training teachers so that *all* teachers can support students regardless of disability status.

Your advocacy becomes crucial if your school district still needs to embrace inclusion fully. You might engage with teachers and administrators to discuss implementing inclusive practices in your child's classroom. If your schedule permits, you can connect with other parents of children with disabilities to share experiences and strategies. Work with like-minded parents to influence district-wide policies on inclusion. Persistent and informed advocacy can significantly change a school or school district's practices and culture.

Your child's disability gives them special rights. In the next chapter, we examine how these rights shape your child's educational experience and impact their day-to-day instruction.

> **Tip for Cultivating Joy:** Create something beautiful with your hands. Working with your hands can provide relaxation, rest, and relief for the mind while allowing the brain to work on problems subconsciously. It is inherently pleasurable and contributes to maintaining a healthy mood. YouTube has tutorials that can help

you learn how to knit, crochet, and needlepoint. You might find joy in gardening, cookie decorating, or other things that require lots of handwork. Dabble with a few of these to find a new hobby to help you find joy during downtime.

Self-Care Tip: If you're anxious, begin a worry list. Your list can be written in a special notepad, saved as a document on your device, or written on a sticky note. Write down any worries you have as they pop into your mind. (This isn't formal! Single words or partial sentences are fine.) Schedule a time to review the list—the following day or on the weekend—and work through the items listed. Until then, let your worries go and know you'll deal with them when you have the mental stamina.

5

Strengthen Learning through Customized Instruction

I learned how to cook by watching Food Network chefs and obsessively reading *Cook's Illustrated*. I hosted my first Thanksgiving in 2009 and have declared it "my" holiday ever since. Some years, our crowd has been larger than others, which means we need to accommodate dietary needs.

In 2015, some extended family joined us. In that group were a cousin who was a vegan and a diabetic family member. To make accommodations for my family, I skipped the academic conference I usually attended the weekend before Thanksgiving and prepared as much food in advance as possible. I was nervous as I prepared for that Thanksgiving for another reason. I had to scrap many of my tried-and-true recipes since I had eliminated gluten from my diet earlier in the year.

Despite the adjustments, I discovered the joy of creating a Thanksgiving feast that catered to everyone's dietary needs. Today, Thanksgiving remains a day of togetherness, showcasing the power of accommodation and modifications to ensure inclusion and shared joy.

Shouldn't education do the same for all of our children?

ACCESSIBILITY VERSUS ACCOMMODATIONS

It would be perfect if schools were accessible to all students. Katie Rose Guest Pryal, JD, PhD, explains, "Accommodations are not accessibility. Accommodations are special exceptions made for one disabled person who has to jump through lots of hoops to get them. On the other hand, accessibility is the creation of a space that is hospitable to and usable by disabled people, no hoops required." I want curriculum, classrooms, and school buildings to be accessible, which means they're designed proactively. When something is inaccessible, the onus is on the disabled person or their caregiver to ask for an accommodation. While accommodations benefit individuals who require them, accessibility has advantages for everyone.

Universal Design for Learning, or UDL, is an educational framework many schools have adopted to design accessible learning environments. UDL seeks to provide all students with equal opportunities to become expert learners who are goal-oriented, motivated, purposeful, and resourceful.

UDL is built on three core principles, often called the three pillars:

- Engagement focuses on motivation and sustained enthusiasm for learning (the "why" of learning).

- Representation involves presenting information and content in various ways to support understanding (the "what" of learning).

- Action and Expression offer students diverse ways to demonstrate their knowledge and skills (the "how" of learning).

UDL changes an environment's design rather than changing the learner. Therefore, it's appropriate to allow schools to accommodate the needs and abilities of all learners. By intentionally designing learning environments, minimizing barriers, and reducing unnecessary hurdles, all learners can be challenged and engaged to maximize learning outcomes.

UDL's guidelines undergird good teaching. However, not all schools have a UDL framework. Therefore, it is necessary to work with your child's teachers and service providers to customize their instruction through interventions, accommodations, modifications, technology use, etc.

In Chapter 1, I provided an overview of MTSS interventions. Typically, extra support and interventions are implemented *before* a school-based evaluation. If an evaluation shows the child has a disability, the conversation shifts to creating an IEP, where students are eligible for specially designed instruction to help them meet their goals.

As you already know from Chapter 3, accommodation is *how* students access their learning and the school environment. A modification is *what* the student is taught or expected to learn. We'll explore the nitty-gritty of those terms in this chapter. But first, it's essential to understand what specially designed instruction is.

UNDERSTANDING SPECIALLY DESIGNED INSTRUCTION

The concept of specially designed instruction, or SDI, addresses the effects of the child's disability, helps them master IEP goals, and ensures access to and progress in the general education curriculum. It involves adapting the following things to meet the *individual* needs of a child with a disability:

- **Content:** *what* the child learns, which is linked to the standards
- **Methodology:** *how* instruction is designed and the teaching methods used
- **Instructional Delivery:** *where/when* instruction is delivered during the school day

SDI is part of IDEA's Sec. 300.39 (b) (3). It states:

Specially designed instruction means adapting, as appropriate to the needs of an eligible child under this part, the content, methodology, or delivery of instruction—

(i) To address the unique needs of the child that result from the child's disability; and

(ii) To ensure access of the child to the general curriculum, so that the child can meet the educational standards within the jurisdiction of the public agency that apply to all children.

Sec. 300.39 (b) (3), *https://sites.ed.gov/idea/regs/b/a/300.39/b/3*

SDI refers to the explicit, deliberately planned instruction that the special educator or other school personnel uses to meet the unique needs of students with disabilities in various areas, such as academics, behavior, and social skills. SDI encompasses various aspects of the student's education, such as materials, techniques, assessments, and activities. SDI addresses a student's unique challenges that arise because of their disability. Thoughtfully designed SDI helps students progress toward their IEP goals while allowing them to access grade-level content that leads to optimal learning outcomes.

Distinguishing SDI from Differentiation, Accommodation, and Modification

SDI is often confused with other terminologies.

- **It is not differentiation.** Differentiation involves tailoring instruction to meet the learning needs of *all* students in a classroom, regardless of their disability status. SDI focuses on providing instruction specially designed for students with disabilities and is tied to an IEP goal. It goes beyond general differentiation by addressing the specific needs of individual students with disabilities.
- **It is not an accommodation.** Accommodation changes the way information is presented or accessed by a student. It is a support or adjustment to help a student with disabilities access the general education curriculum. While accommodations can be part of SDI, SDI encompasses more comprehensive instructional strategies beyond simple accommodations.
- **It is not a modification.** Modifications change the curriculum or content that a student is expected to learn. It typically involves altering the material's complexity, depth, or breadth. SDI focuses on providing instructional methods and techniques tailored to meet a student's particular learning needs without necessarily changing the content.

Delivering and Integrating SDI

All students with an IEP must have SDI. The essential things to understand about SDI are:

- A licensed special educator or related service provider (such as a speech therapist) delivers instruction in or out of the general education classroom.
- It is designed expressly for your child's needs.
- It does not modify the curriculum by lowering standards or expectations.
- It is provided to a child at no cost.

SDI helps students keep up with their grade-level peers by giving them extra support in areas related to their disability. This support could include explaining things differently, reteaching using special tools or materials, or chunking assignments so the easiest step is completed first. The goal is for your child to be in the general education classroom whenever possible, learning alongside their classmates. SDI helps them succeed in that environment.

SDIs should be unique to each student and necessary for them to achieve their educational goals. (If support or accommodation is available to all students, it should not be considered SDI because it is not truly *specially designed.*) The sign of effective SDI is seeing a child make satisfactory progress on their IEP goal(s).

Some districts have master lists of accommodations, supports, and strategies from which teachers and service providers can choose when preparing an IEP. While these lists are a time-saver for educators, you don't want your child's IEP to contain many items dragged and dropped into the document without considering your child's *specific* needs.

Ideally, the general education teacher, special education teacher, and related service providers should discuss the SDI they can implement to help your child meet their IEP goals as they're creating an IEP. As a parent, you may ask questions at the IEP meeting to better understand why certain SDI is suggested for your child.

Speak up if you think something from the proposed SDI needs to be added. As a member of the IEP team, you can suggest supports you'd like the team to consider if you think other things might help your child.

CUSTOMIZING INSTRUCTION IN PRACTICE

Let's look at several illustrated instances of how the learning environment was tailored for children. You might see aspects of your child in some of these descriptive examples. I hope these examples help you better understand how a child's learning environment is customized.

Important Note: In the vignettes that follow, some of the language may include terms that are outdated or not aligned with current inclusive practices; these examples reflect terminology still used in some educational settings. Using these terms is not an endorsement of such language but a reflection of existing institutional norms.

Academics

Will is a fourth grader who qualified for an IEP due to a specific learning disability related to reading. His initial IEP had some of the following items listed under SDI and modifications:

- Provide small-group, direct instruction using a multisensory, research-based reading program with frequent opportunities for repetition and review of learned skills.

- Pair written/visual directions with oral directions.

- Provide audiobooks and text-to-speech versions of articles and short stories.

- Read tests aloud when reading comprehension isn't being assessed.

- Provide instructions using the accessibility features on the iPad.

- Use an easy-to-read font (Arial, Helvetica) on handouts and texts.

- Decrease visual input on the page when doing classwork by covering portions with blank paper and/or using a reading guide (like a ruler, line marker, or index card) to assist with attending to reading a line at a time.

Will was pulled out of his classroom during the station rotations. He despised leaving his classroom to work on reading since it made him feel "like a dummy" while the rest of his friends stayed there for the entire reading period. Often, Will refused to go to the learning support classroom. When Will went to learning support, he was usually disengaged and put his head on the table. One time, he even fell asleep!

Will's case manager was also the special educator who pulled Will out of class to work in his classroom. He talked with Will to see how he could incentivize him to not only show up but also put effort into doing the work. Will, an affable kid, told him nothing would make him do the work unless he was in his own classroom.

Frustrated by Will's obstinacy and the time he was taking away from other students' learning, the case manager spoke with his building principal, who brought in the special education supervisor to figure things out. They asked Will's case manager to consider doing small-group work inside his classroom instead of the learning support room. Since this would impact two other students (in that they'd receive their services alongside Will in his classroom, not the learning support room), the principal put feelers out to the other parents to see if this would be acceptable to them. After the other parents consented, an IEP meeting with Will's dad was called. It was proposed that the specialized reading instruction be implemented in Will's general education classroom during station rotation time. Even though Will wouldn't rotate to different stations, he'd be *in* his classroom to receive reading support. Will's dad said he'd sign off on an IEP revision that changed the location of reading support services if Will agreed to try this out.

While Will's case manager disliked uprooting himself to Will's classroom, he wanted to try out a push-in model. Within a week, Will's case manager found a way to help Will engage with the work without feeling humiliated by having to change classrooms. Will was attentive and participated fully in all the reading instruction his case manager delivered inside his classroom.

Penny has articulation issues and dysfluent speech (sometimes called *stuttering*), which qualified her for an IEP due to a speech and language impairment. While she made substantial progress since her initial diagnosis, she grew frustrated with looking and sounding different from her peers in sixth grade. Her astute sixth-grade teacher consulted with Penny's mother, her SLP, and her school's technology integration coach since she was worried about Penny losing confidence in her academic abilities.

The IEP team invited Penny to join the meeting so she could share what was working for her and what was frustrating her. During the meeting, Penny admitted that she would rather hunt and peck at the keys than use the speech-to-text feature on her school-issued tablet since she found she had to enunciate her words dramatically for it to pick up what she was saying correctly. She also stated that she hated getting called on unexpectedly in class or giving a presentation in front of the entire class.

The technology integration coach suggested a typing program to teach Penny keyboarding skills since her typing speed was slow. Second, she would provide Penny with instruction on how to use the pronunciation feature on her device, which would allow her to train the tablet to understand words the way Penny said them (for instance, teaching the device that when she said *duh,* it needed to spell that as *the*). Finally, the tech coach scheduled a weekly check-in meeting with Penny to help her with any technical issues with speech-to-text or typing.

Penny already had several SDIs in her IEP that addressed articulation issues. They were:

- Model targeted speech sounds with repeated opportunities for practice

- Use verbal, visual, and tactile prompts to assist Penny in achieving proper articulatory placement for targeted speech sounds

- Use minimal-pairs instruction to emphasize the different auditory and oral features of sounds targeted in therapy

Her SLP suggested some new SDI for Penny based on her concerns. Moving forward, Penny's classroom and specials teachers would:

- Provide Penny with extra time to formulate her thoughts for oral tasks

- Preselect the questions Penny would answer aloud so she could rehearse her answers

- Avoid asking multiple questions in quick succession to reduce speaking demands

- Allow Penny to record her oral presentations on video in a setting where she feels most comfortable speaking

By springtime, Penny had improved her speech-to-text and keyboarding skills, thanks to the support from the tech coach. She took a brave step two months after the IEP meeting when she decided to try an oral presentation in front of her classmates. She said, "Sometimes my speech gets bumpy, and I might repeat myself. Please be patient with me while I work through it." When she finished presenting, her classmates cheered for her, which increased her confidence and made her opt to prerecord oral presentations only when she was less comfortable with the content. While Penny would still need school-based speech therapy in middle school, and the SDI would stay in place, she was better positioned to handle the rigors of speaking in front of her peers upon graduation from sixth grade.

Behavior

Robby was performing above his fourth-grade level when he could attend to tasks. He had received an IEP in second grade under "other health impairment" because his ADHD diagnosis created a need for help with attention and focus. When he returned from summer vacation, Robby began leaving the classroom unannounced, melting down when faced with timed, on-demand writing assessments, and screaming or crying (which could be heard down the hall, disrupting many students) when he became upset.

Robby's teacher was frustrated, and Robby's case manager was exhausted since he was shirking his responsibilities to his other students to attend to Robby daily. Therefore, Robby's case manager called an IEP meeting to determine whether a functional behavioral assessment, or FBA, could be done to help them figure out three things:

1. What causes Robby to act out?
2. Why does Robby behave disruptively?
3. How could teachers help Robby stay focused and not disturb others?

The team, which included Robby's parents, agreed to the FBA. Once the FBA was completed, the team learned the following:

- Robby's meltdowns were usually caused by task avoidance, specifically during a transition to writing workshop or before an on-demand assessment. If he cried or screamed in the classroom, he'd be removed from the classroom to calm down, which allowed him to miss writing. He also wouldn't have to complete an on-demand writing assessment if he eloped from the classroom moments before an assessment since adults would spend time helping him calm down outside the classroom.

- Sometimes there wasn't a significant trigger for Robby's meltdowns. For example, some of his meltdowns were caused by minor issues like his pencil falling on the floor or walking into a table. It was noted that when Robby became distraught over a seemingly minor incident, he would yell but not shed any tears.

Once Robby's FBA report was reviewed, a behavior intervention plan, or BIP, was created to help minimize his meltdowns. (A BIP is similar to a positive behavior support plan, or PBSP. However, a BIP is often recognized as a legal document in educational settings.) First, Robby would be given three break cards per day. Robby was taught to hand the teacher a break card calmly whenever his stress level increased. Next, he was instructed to walk down the hall to the resource room without yelling. From there, he'd sit on a beanbag chair to collect himself using calming strategies taught to him by the guidance counselor. Robby did not receive any acknowledgment of his presence until five minutes passed *or* he was calm. From there, his case manager or the school psychologist would help Robby solve the problem and return him to class.

Second, Robby was reassigned to the resource room to take future on-demand writing assessments so he would have emotional support. Upon entry, one of the teachers or paraeducators in the room would express confidence in his abilities. If Robby felt frustrated, he could take a short break within the resource room where he'd receive more encouraging words.

As for daily writing workshops, a paraeducator swung by Robby's classroom five minutes before writing time to provide him with a planned break, which usually included rolling on an exercise ball or doing wall push-ups in the school's sensory break room. Upon reentering the classroom, Robby's teacher shared the writing skill or strategy they'd be working on and delivered a positive affirmation about his ability to write well. In addition, his classroom teacher checked Robby's progress within five minutes of the end of each writing minilesson. Robby was a writer who was approaching grade-level benchmarks in writing, but detested the subject and lacked confidence that what he had to say was "good." His teacher affirmed Robby's ability to complete the day's work independently. If a strategy was tricky, Robby would be pulled into a small group with his teacher for support.

Once Robby's team understood his triggers and implemented these supports, they noticed he stayed calm and was in the classroom more frequently than he was out. There were setbacks, such as Robby pushing a student who teased him for being scared to complete an on-demand writing assessment, but overall the meltdowns decreased. As Robby moved to fifth grade, his next teacher continued the BIP, so Robby would receive up to three breaks a day and would leave the room for all timed writing assessments. By the middle of fifth grade, he was able to make it through the week with just a planned break right before writing workshop. He thrived in fifth grade thanks to how the school staff responded to Robby's behavioral issues.

Eliza received an IEP under the emotional disability category. (The official term used in IDEA is *emotional disturbance*. Often, the word *disability* is used instead of *disturbance* to destigmatize mental health issues.) A family member had abused her at a young age. She was anxious, at times used aggressive language toward classmates, and acted out frequently in class. Toward the end of third grade, she became enraged when her teacher called the main office and asked someone to pick her up after she had made inappropriate comments to another student. When the school secretary showed up, Eliza kicked her in the shins and ran to the cafeteria. The situation escalated quickly, and by the end of the episode, the assistant principal and school psychologist had been punched by Eliza.

After disciplinary action was taken, and a transfer to a more restrictive classroom was rejected, Eliza's IEP team met to make a plan for fourth grade. They placed Eliza in a highly structured classroom with a kind but firm teacher who already had a calm-down space in her classroom, taught and practiced routines, and successfully used check-in/check-out sheets (described in Chapter 7).

Eliza's aunt was her caregiver and knew Eliza needed help but wanted her in the general education setting as much as possible. The IEP team suggested that Eliza receive small-group instruction in social skills for 20 minutes daily. In addition, she received counseling sessions once a week. The following SDI was added to Eliza's IEP:

- Explicitly teach conflict resolution and anger management techniques.
- Teach and practice coping skills and calm-down techniques.
- Provide positive reinforcement for appropriate behaviors.
- Teach strategies for recognizing physical symptoms of emotions.

With the addition of supports and services, Eliza learned valuable coping and self-regulation skills and was less verbally aggressive. Her fourth-grade teacher worked diligently to establish a positive relationship with her from the first day of school. Eliza became dysregulated outside of the classroom in the cafeteria and with her related arts and PE teachers. Since Eliza wanted to please her classroom teacher, her teacher would talk to Eliza privately about any reports she received from outside the classroom, especially if a referral to the main office was threatened. By the end of fourth grade, Eliza progressed toward her IEP goals and experienced more success with her peers. While she still required accommodations, supports, and services, Eliza learned how to manage her anger, be more at ease with her peers and teachers, and feel like a valued classroom community member.

Social-Emotional

Xavier is a fifth-grade student whose primary disability category is autism spectrum. While Xavier has some sensory issues, his previous teachers found accommodations that worked for him within the classroom environment, such as:

- Availability of a lower stimulation work area for times when visual or auditory input may impact self-regulation
- Use of headphones to support self-regulation in noisy environments
- Preferential seating with lower visual distractions (for example, using a cardboard divider as an "office" when needed)

By fifth grade, Xavier's most significant challenge was social pragmatics, which includes taking turns in a conversation, understanding the implied meaning of a message, and comprehending nonverbal cues. Lacking proper use of social language meant that Xavier struggled with cooperative group work, making friends, and having conversations that included circles of communication. While Xavier received direct instruction to address social interactions with a small group of students once a week in the resource room, he wasn't progressing toward IEP goals to improve his pragmatic language skills.

Xavier's family was concerned about his pragmatic language challenges at home and contacted the school to see if they impacted him in the classroom. They requested that the IEP team convene. Once the team met, the special educator providing social skills training shared progress-monitoring data that illustrated Xavier wasn't making sufficient progress toward his goals. Xavier's grandparents, his primary caregivers, were frustrated and asked if he could receive more social skills instruction since he was struggling at home and in the community.

First, the team decided Xavier needed to be paired with a different group of kids to work on social skills *twice* a week since it seemed the members of his once-a-week social skills group had different challenges than Xavier. Second, the school's SLP was invited to sit in on the meeting (because Xavier was on his caseload through the end of second grade). The SLP suggested adding Xavier back to his caseload to support him by adding speech-language goals, modeling skills, and providing repeated opportunities for practice.

In addition, the following were added to the SDI and Modification section in Xavier's IEP:

- Avoiding nonliteral language or forms of speech, such as sarcasm, idioms, and/or metaphors, unless formally taught
- Providing small-group, direct instruction with repeated opportunities to practice circles of communication
- Using a research-based curriculum, small-group, direct instruction to address social interactions and perspective taking

Xavier's grandparents were satisfied with this proposal but asked to hold an informal meeting a month later.

When the IEP team reconvened, Xavier's grandparents brought an advocate since they remained skeptical. They needed someone not emotionally invested in the situation to be a third voice in the room and help Xavier get what he needed. It was shown that Xavier was progressing with his new social skills group and even began playing with some of the kids in his social skills group at recess. The SLP reported that Xavier was showing up to sessions and was willing to work and communicate with his peers, but he didn't have enough progress-monitoring data to show growth.

The advocate spoke up and asked what else could be done to help Xavier outside the resource and therapy rooms. The assistant principal, the LEA representative at the meeting, suggested having Xavier join a lunch bunch run by the school counselor twice a week. All students in that group were in fourth grade but faced similar pragmatic language challenges. Therefore, the school counselor worked on skills like taking turns in conversations and understanding jokes and sarcasm. When the advocate asked why this lunch group wasn't offered to Xavier sooner, the case manager said it wasn't considered because the students were one year younger than Xavier. Xavier's grandparents didn't mind the slight age gap and requested that Xavier join the lunch group twice a week rather than eat in the cafeteria.

The advocate requested that the IEP team be reconvened in two months to allow ample time for progress-monitoring data to be collected. At that meeting, the SLP, guidance counselor, and special education teacher shared their data, showing gains with the items they monitored. Xavier's grandparents said they noticed some progress at home but not when they went to church. The case manager stated that since some progress was being made, the SDI was working and they should stay the course rather than make any additional changes that would increase the amount of time Xavier spent receiving special education supports and services. Given that Xavier had one more school year until middle school, Xavier's grandparents agreed to this plan.

By the middle of sixth grade, Xavier was doing better with cooperative group work since he had learned to take turns in conversations. Everyone on the team noticed he was beginning to understand nonliteral language, progressing toward understanding words with multiple meanings, and being in on jokes. His grandparents reported that he had made two friends and sometimes did things with them on the weekends. While Xavier still needed support and services, growth was occurring, for which his grandparents were thankful.

Amelia had a variety of developmental delays during the first years of her life. Walking and talking late, Amelia spent a lot of time in occupational, physical, and speech therapy. Due to a variety of parental concerns, Amelia had genetic testing done and was diagnosed with Kleefstra syndrome, which is a genetic condition that presented in Amelia as communication delays, an intellectual disability, autism, low muscle tone, and gastrointestinal problems. As a result, she attended a special preschool for children with disabilities. By kindergarten, Amelia's parents opted to send her to a public school.

Educating Amelia in the general education classroom wasn't possible when she entered kindergarten due to her high support needs. From a hygiene perspective alone, Amelia needed to be in a smaller classroom with a private, safe space where an adult could assist her with toileting. By second grade, Amelia was independent and used the bathroom, so her family asked if Amelia could spend more time with her same-age peers in the general education setting since they didn't want Amelia isolated in the same small classroom where she received instruction all day.

The school suggested starting with lunch and art, music, and physical education. Being with the general population was good for Amelia since it allowed her to practice socialization. To make this happen, Amelia, who had a paraeducator working with her and two other children, was accompanied to the special classes to ensure Amelia had extra support.

Amelia received training—from her special education teacher in a social skills group and from her speech therapist during small-group sessions—for engaging with other students in circles of communication to improve her conversational skills. A paraeducator was present with Amelia during lunch and specials to assist with engaging conversation prompts and encouragement when speaking with her peers. Twice a week Amelia participated in a snack bunch, an adult-supported peer group run by the guidance counselor and the speech therapist, who modeled how to socialize during snack time.

As Amelia settled into third grade, she required less support from the paraeducator since she continued working on circles of communication in social skills and speech therapy. Plus, she went to a third-grade general education classroom for morning meetings three days a week. Attending the morning meeting helped her become more familiar with the other students. It helped her learn how to engage with her same-age peers in another setting supported by the general education teacher.

MOVING TOWARD ACCESS

After a decade of gluten-free living, I've learned to eat ahead of time and stash a granola bar in my purse when invited to a party. Well-meaning hosts try to accommodate by asking if invitees have dietary restrictions on a reply card, but I've learned there may be only a handful of things I can eat.

Imagine my surprise when I walked into a wedding reception last year, and the groom's mother pulled me aside to walk me down the buffet line. Despite labels that stated what was gluten-free, she made sure I knew what my safe options were ahead of time. It was the first reception I've been to in a long time where I truly felt confident with every bite of food in my mouth. In the same way that my 2015 Thanksgiving menu provided options for everyone in every course, the gracious hosts of this wedding provided me with *access* from appetizers to dessert. I left the reception with a full belly, a full heart, and a purse of uneaten granola bars.

I want kids with IEPs to feel as cared for and seen as I did when the groom's mother walked me through that buffet line. Truly customized instruction helps students with IEPs access the general education curriculum and nonacademic activities that are part of the school community. When the right things are in place, children feel seen, valued, and heard.

Now that you're familiar with the components of SDI and have seen how six student IEP teams have worked to help students reach their IEP goals, you're ready to prepare for IEP meetings.

Tip for Cultivating Joy: In the poem "A Lazy Thought" by Eve Merriam, she says it takes a lot of slow to grow. There are endless comparisons between plant growth and the rest of life. Therefore, get gardening or growing with your child. Visit a local nursery to get some seeds, herbs, vegetables, succulents, or whatever you and your child can commit to nurturing together. Discuss the time it takes to nurture and grow whatever you choose. Help your child see how growth happens over time, not all at once.

Self-Care Tip: Say yes the next time a friend or family member offers to help you with an errand or to provide respite care. In *The Amen Effect: Ancient Wisdom to Mend Our Broken Hearts and the World,* Sharon Brous asserts, "It's an act of self-love, to let someone else take your hand and lift you up, especially if you are used to doing the heavy lifting yourself." This may be the season of your life when you need to receive help. At some point, you'll be able to offer a helping hand to someone else.

6

Prepare, Partner, and Advocate for IEP Meeting Success

I want to be real with you. To this day, I get the jitters before some IEP meetings. Being on the other side (the parent side rather than the teacher side) means there's more at stake because we will discuss *my* kid in the IEP meeting! Over the years, I've found I can calm my nerves to a low hum if I overprepare, hydrate, and listen to classical music before the meeting.

Just as classical music isn't everyone's jam, not everyone needs to overprepare for a meeting. But it helps to do some preparation so you can collaborate effectively with your child's school.

You've heard it several times, but it's worth repeating: *You* are your child's first teacher. You know your child best. You have the expertise *the team needs* to help your child reach their fullest potential. This makes you an integral part of the IEP team!

It's easy to feel overwhelmed when you walk into an IEP meeting, especially by yourself. Many adults sit around the table, so it often resembles a board meeting rather than a meeting about a young child. While some might be familiar faces, you may also meet adults you've never seen. Unless you're a gregarious person with the confidence of a pageant contestant (of which I am neither), you might feel some jitters.

This chapter will help you prepare for and get through IEP meetings. It will also provide you with ways to monitor your child's progress between meetings.

GATHER INFORMATION

Gathering everything you'll need a week before the meeting is essential to decrease the frazzled or anxious feelings that manifest in many people before IEP meetings:

- Request all relevant assessments, documents, and reports be shared with you *as far ahead of the meeting as possible.* Ensure you've read through them. Flag anything unclear to you, items you wish to discuss further in the meeting, and concerns about anything you receive before the meeting.

- Request an IEP Glossary. Many schools have glossaries of terms commonly used in special education. This can help you decipher educational jargon and acronyms.

- Prepare and share a list of issues you want to discuss and/or specific questions you have for the IEP team. It helps to share these lists beforehand so the team can be prepared to respond to your concerns during the meeting.

- Create a list of observations, concerns, and/or progress you've noticed at home or in the community. Your lists can be typed up or scribbled on sticky notes. Whatever works for you! This information might be helpful to the team's discussion, so having it in front of you would be useful.

- Bring any external evaluations or reports to the meeting. You can also share these documents with school personnel ahead of time. The more information the IEP team has about your child, the better they can respond to your child's needs.

- Create an informational sheet about your child that you can share at your child's initial or annual IEP meetings. (You might call it a "Things You Need to Know About _____" sheet, an FAQ sheet, or a parent vision statement. See Chapter 7 for a blank form you can adapt for your own use, plus a filled-in example. You can also download the blank form at *www.guilford.com/shubitz-materials.*) Include a recent photo of your child on the sheet. A sheet like this personalizes your child, so they aren't just another kid with an IEP.

Establishing Rapport with the Classroom Teacher

You and your child's classroom teacher have the deepest insight of your child. If you're feeling uneasy about an upcoming meeting, ask your child's teacher if you can chat over the phone. Most teachers I've worked with are compassionate people who can help you prepare for a meeting by explaining who will be there and what will be discussed.

RESPOND TO THE INVITATION

After your child has an IEP, you will meet with the IEP team for an annual IEP meeting. As a parent, *you can call the IEP team together for a meeting at any time.* These can be regularly scheduled check-in meetings (for instance, at the end of each marking period) or random meetings to discuss a concern or to touch base about a specific issue.

Before the meeting, you will receive an invitation to participate in the IEP meeting. On that form, it will state the purpose of the meeting (typically for planning and placement), the invited team members, and the meeting's location. Then, there will be a section for you to respond. You will state whether or not you will attend the meeting. If the time or location of the meeting is not convenient, you'll suggest an alternate date on that form. In addition, *you* can request accommodations, such as needing an interpreter, wheelchair access, meeting documents in an accessible format, or a virtual meeting if you cannot make it to the school physically at the proposed time.

Sign and return the invitation as soon as possible to reserve your time slot. Notify the school if you plan to bring along an advocate, a family member not listed on the invitation, or a friend who will take notes.

Will Your Child Attend the Meeting?

Transition and postsecondary planning begins once students turn 16 (or younger in many states). At this point, your child will be invited to attend the IEP meeting. While it isn't required by law for your elementary school child to attend their IEP meeting, you might consider having them there for *part* of the meeting. Not only does this make your child three-dimensional, but it also allows your child to begin to understand their IEP so they can learn how to advocate for themselves.

UNDERSTAND YOUR RIGHTS

You'll receive a copy of the procedural safeguards notice at or before every IEP meeting. It is a dense, boring read, but it's also important!

As the Introduction mentioned, legal protections are afforded to your child from ages 3 to 21 by the Individuals with Disabilities Education Act (IDEA). These legal protections are referred to as *procedural safeguards*. School districts provide parents with a list of procedural safeguards that inform you of your rights and your child's rights under IDEA. Typically, schools will provide this to you in writing once a year at your child's annual IEP meeting. However, if you call a meeting to touch base with your child's team, this is another time you'll be handed a copy of the procedural safeguards so you know what your rights are.

I didn't read the boring procedural safeguards booklet cover to cover until my child was in upper elementary school, which meant I was flying by the seat of my pants. I don't recommend this kind of on-the-job learning! I encourage you to familiarize yourself with these safeguards *before* the meeting. (You can find your state's version of the procedural safeguards with a quick Google search, such as *Procedural Safeguards Colorado*.) At a bare minimum, read through the table of contents and peruse the sections you believe will apply to you. Then save a copy on your mobile device and computer so you can pull it up anytime.

Reevaluations

School districts are required to do a triennial evaluation. Your child will be reevaluated to see if their needs have changed and if they still qualify for special education services for their disability. You may request a reevaluation sooner if you see a need. Under IDEA, your child can be reevaluated annually. However, since the process is time-consuming, you should have a substantial reason to request more frequent reevaluations.

KNOW THE FLOW: THE ANNUAL MEETING

Every annual IEP meeting will be run differently since every school district has its own style. Given my experiences as a teacher and parent, here's how most annual planning and placement meetings unfold:

- **Welcome and Introductions:** Typically, meetings begin with the case manager welcoming everyone to the meeting and introducing all of the people present in the room. If a time limit or constraint is in place, this will be shared with you so you'll know approximately how long the meeting will last.

- **Review of Present Levels:** The team will review your child's present levels, discussing your child's strengths and areas for growth based on their assessments, grades, and observations (see the box below). The present levels can cover academic achievement and functional performance, which includes, but isn't limited to, behavior, communication, mobility, and social skills.

Many school psychologists, teachers, and related service providers will provide an opportunity to rephrase and paraphrase the information from the assessments or other data they present. Some people might start using parent-friendly language, while others will ask if you have questions as or after they present information to you.

Present Levels Matter

1. **Establishing a Baseline:** Present levels are a snapshot of your child's current skills.
2. **Setting Clear Objectives:** This baseline is the starting point for writing objectives and measuring yearly growth.
3. **Tracking Progress:** Measuring improvement accurately is impossible without a clear starting point.

To use a sports analogy, swimmers need to know their current 50-meter time for each stroke to set specific goals and track their improvement. Saying they're "pretty good" at swimming backstroke isn't specific enough. Swimmers can't improve what they don't measure, so they do time trials before a season begins. This helps them determine how much they're progressing during the season.

- **Progress Review and Goal Setting:** The heart of the meeting will be a discussion of IEP goals. You'll have the opportunity to examine data to see how your child progressed toward the goals of the previous IEP. You'll learn whether or not goals were met, which will help the team decide whether to adjust them. Based on the review of your child's progress, new goals and objectives will be developed for the upcoming 12-month period. The goals will be written in specific, measurable, attainable, results-oriented, and time-based, or SMART, ways and will be monitored throughout the year.

- **Determination of Services and Supports:** You'll review your child's services, including a discussion about their current supports and whether or not additional supports and services are needed. The conversation about services can discuss any adjustments your child needs or additional resources that should be considered. Anything that could enhance your child's success (such as assistive technology, door-to-door transportation, or specialized equipment) will be discussed.

- This part of the meeting also includes a discussion of specially designed instruction (see Chapter 5).

- **Extended School Year, or ESY:** ESY is a specialized education service for students with disabilities, provided as part of their IEP to prevent skill regression during breaks. The IEP team determines eligibility annually based on the child's needs and potential recoupment difficulties. ESY offers free instruction and services focused on specific IEP goals, unlike summer school.

- **Placement Considerations** (if applicable): Your child's current educational placement might be discussed to determine if it continues to be the best fit. Chapter 4 mentions that the least restrictive environment, or LRE, can change during the day based on instruction and settings. The team must prioritize the child's inclusion alongside nondisabled children.

TIP Some school districts will build in time to ask questions at the beginning of the meeting. Remember, you can ask questions *at any point* during the meeting. See the box on pages 106–107 for sample questions.

- **Parental Questions, Concerns, and Input:** This is a chance to ask questions or raise concerns before the case manager adjourns the meeting. If you wish to discuss more and time doesn't permit, you may ask to reconvene at another mutually convenient time. (You may request an informal meeting with school personnel once a Notice of Recommended Educational Placement/Prior Written Notice, or NOREP/PWN, is issued to you after the meeting.)

- **Next Steps and Closing:** The case manager usually summarizes the meeting and outlines the actions each team member will be responsible for. If a time constraint leaves the discussion incomplete, another time might be set to finish it before the meeting is adjourned.

Sample Questions to Ask during an Annual IEP Meeting

Curriculum and Academic Progress

- What does my child need to be successful with the general education curriculum?
- How has my child progressed academically and socially since the last IEP meeting?
- What adjustments need to be made to the current IEP to better support my child's learning and development?

Strengths and Support Needs

- What are my child's strengths, and how can we leverage them?
- What areas does my child still need support in?
- What programmatic changes or approaches need to be adjusted if my child's support needs aren't being met?

Accommodations and Services

- Can you show me how often the accommodations are used and whether they are effective?
- What does that SDI mean, and how is it accomplished daily?
- Can you explain what services and supports will be provided to help my child reach their goals? Who will be providing these services, and how often?
- What is the provider's training and experience working with children who have similar needs?

Progress Monitoring and Independence

- How will my child's progress be monitored? How often will I receive updates?
- What are you doing to increase my child's independence to do _____ without your support in the future? What's next?

Home and Community Support

- Can you recommend strategies or resources for me to support my child's IEP goals?
- Are there any community resources or organizations that can provide additional support for my child and our family?

Communication and Future Planning

- What's the best method of communication (such as email, text, phone, or learning management system) for me to follow up with you when I have questions?
- Will there be any transitions or changes in my child's educational program that I should be aware of?

Additional IEP Meetings

There are many reasons you might meet between annual IEP meetings (see the table below). Therefore, the flow of each meeting will be determined by the case manager, who will set the agenda.

Typical Kinds of IEP Meetings

Review and Revise Meeting	Make adjustments to your child's IEP. You may discuss your child's: • academic progress or decline • functional needs • social and emotional needs
Disciplinary Meeting	Determine if your child should be suspended or expelled for a behavioral issue. This meeting determines if their behavior is related to their disability.
Reevaluation Meeting	Reassesses your child to determine if they continue to qualify for special education services.
Dismissal Meeting	Review your child's progress when they've met their goals and no longer need special education services.

In addition, you may call an informal meeting to discuss concerns or adjustments that need to be made. You might meet at a predetermined time (such as monthly or at the end of a marking period) to discuss how things are going at school and/or at home. To use time effectively, you should reach out to your child's case manager beforehand to share your concerns and why you wish to reconvene.

COMMON PROBLEMS AT IEP MEETINGS

Sometimes parents feel their attendance at an IEP meeting is allowed solely out of a sense of obligation. The school invites them, and they must attend so their child can continue receiving services and support. Other times, parents feel disregarded by school officials, as though they're not even in the room. Sometimes parents have been made to feel they did something wrong since "their child" is misbehaving or not meeting their goals. Anything that makes you feel like less than a VIP member of the IEP team is problematic and needs to be addressed.

You've already read about the importance of preparation and knowing your rights. Let's look at possible issues that can occur during an IEP meeting and tips to help you navigate these challenges.

Feeling Uninformed

Even if you've prepared for the meeting by requesting and reading the documents, you may feel uninformed. IEP meetings can be full of educational jargon and processes. As a parent, you may feel overwhelmed by all the information or unsure of what questions to ask.

- **Ask for explanations:** If a term or concept is confusing, politely ask the team to explain it further.
- **Focus on understanding the impact:** Don't get bogged down in jargon, concentrate on how the IEP will impact your child's education.

Disagreements with the Team

Sometimes you may disagree with the school's assessment of your child's needs or the proposed goals and services.

- **Communicate your concerns:** Aim to speak up *in the moment* about an issue, service, or support directly impacting your child. Use a professional, respectful tone and voice your concern.

- **Ask for data:** The school must have objective data to remove things from an IEP. Have the team share and explain any data they have to help you better understand their position.

Pressure to Accept the IEP as Presented

IEP meetings can feel rushed, leaving parents to feel pressured to accept the IEP as is without fully understanding it or addressing their concerns.

- **Be assertive, not aggressive:** Communicate your concerns about the IEP directly.

- **Ask for more time if you need to mull things over:** Use "think time" to formulate more questions and talk to friends you trust or an advocate.

- **Just say no:** If you object to the proposed IEP, you can request an informal meeting, mediation, or a due process hearing. Be sure to invoke the "stay put" rights, which vary by state but are guaranteed under Sec. 300.518 of IDEA, so your child's supports and services remain in place while you and the school work things out. (See Resources.)

- **One signature:** You must sign only the attendance sheet at the IEP meeting. That's it!

Lack of Communication or Collaboration

Ideally, IEP meetings are a collaborative effort. However, you may feel the school team isn't listening to your input or is not open to considering your suggestions.

- **Ask specific questions:** Instead of making a complaint, ask targeted questions to be more involved in decision making.

- **Focus on shared goals:** Frame the conversation around what's best for your child's success. Emphasize your willingness to work together.

- **Find a parent advocate:** Ask to reconvene soon to allow yourself time to find an advocate who can help you navigate communication challenges and ensure your voice is heard. You can often find phone numbers for advocacy organizations in your state at the back of the procedural safeguards notice. (See Resources.)

Power Imbalance

You might feel intimidated by the professionals in the room.

- **Don't be afraid to ask questions:** Put school personnel to work for you and ask questions whenever you feel unsure. Don't worry about how you'll be perceived. They're the experts, and it's their job to make things understandable so you can properly advocate for your child.

- **Remember your power:** Due to your relationship, you have a unique perspective and insights into your child that no one else on the IEP team could possibly have. Harness this power by helping the team understand who your child is and how they function at home, if it's vastly different from what they see at school.

Mix of Emotions

Many IEP meetings can be emotionally charged, especially if you feel your child's needs aren't being met.

- **Communicate your feelings:** If you feel safe sharing, explain your feelings to the team. Explain your hope for your child's success and your frustration with aspects of the process, their progress, and so on.

- **Take along a support person:** Consider having a trusted friend or family member attend the meeting as a human security blanket. Having someone by your side, observing what you are living through, can help you get another perspective on what transpires and how to move forward after the meeting.

- **Try not to cry:** Do whatever you can to avoid shedding tears at the IEP meeting, even if that means asking for a break to use the restroom so you can collect yourself. While this isn't a business meeting, *it's a business meeting*. Stay strong, and know you can let the waterworks happen after the meeting.

BEYOND THE MEETING

You're an integral part of your child's IEP team, so you must stay involved and keep tabs on what's happening with them in school. Every parent hopes that things will go smoothly and the school-based members of your child's IEP team will ensure your child gets what they need.

I've worked alongside teachers since 2004, and even the most well-intentioned teachers cannot stay on top of everything. Class sizes are too large in most American public schools, so your child might be one of several students with higher support needs. Therefore, you must do your part to keep track of what's happening at school with your child. At times, you may need to be the squeaky wheel, ensuring your child's needs aren't overlooked.

Learning management systems, like Schoology and Seesaw, and school communication tools, such as Parent Square and Remind, keep you informed about what is happening in the classroom. However, individual teachers use these tools differently. Therefore, it's important to find ways to communicate with your child's teachers and service providers if these e-tools don't provide you with enough understanding or access to your child's progress.

Keep the IEP Close at Hand

Many schools will provide you with a hard copy of your child's IEP after you've thoroughly reviewed it and signed the NOREP/PWN paperwork. I find having an electronic copy of the IEP to save on my computer and other digital devices is helpful. This gives me easy access to it wherever and whenever I need it.

You might want to highlight the following sections to keep them at the top of your mind throughout the year.

- **Specially Designed Instruction:** Often children with IEPs have a long list of adaptations, accommodations, modifications, and supplementary aids written into their IEP. If appropriate, make your child aware of what is on this list so they know what they can expect. If your child is an accurate reporter (many aren't in elementary school), you can ask them how it's going, how often they receive certain accommodations, and so on. In addition, you can ask your child's teacher(s) how specific accommodations are working. If your child comes home from school with strong emotions, this is a good time to check in to ensure that specially designed instruction is being carried out.

- **Goals:** At the end of each marking period or semester, you'll most likely receive a progress-monitoring report about your child's goals and their report card. Know the goals your child is working toward so you can use them as a lens to notice progress or regressions. Also, ensure that your child knows their goals in *kid-friendly language* whenever possible.

- **Related Services:** Find out when your child receives their related services. The reason is twofold. First, you want to ensure you don't schedule outside appointments during these times. More importantly, you might want to ask your child what they worked on during a session if you know when they see their related service providers. (It's an example of a more pointed way to learn about your child's day other than generally asking, "How was your day?") If you notice their mood is different—good or bad—on days they receive services, you might discuss this with the providers.

- **Educational Placement:** This section of the IEP helps you understand where (such as general education vs. special education classroom) your child will spend their day. It informs you about the breakdown of their special education services. If your child tells you they're being pulled out of their classroom more or less often than their IEP states they should be, this is a reason to contact your child's case manager to determine what's happening and why.

An IEP is a fluid document. Nothing is set in stone. Something that isn't working can be changed *during* the school year. You may reconvene the IEP team at any time if something feels off. But remember to always start with your child's teacher or case manager to learn more.

YOU ARE READY!

IEP meetings can be overwhelming, so it's important to be prepared and know your rights. Consider your child's needs before the meeting so you are prepared with questions and concerns. Request any relevant documents and assessments. Remember, your input is valuable, so use your voice to advocate for your child year-round.

Tip for Cultivating Joy: Get your mind off an upcoming meeting and make some memories. Select a day when you and your child mutually agree on a location for a day trip. Visit a local farm to pick berries. Go for a hike or a swim at a local, state, or national park. Take in a festival with kid-related activities in a nearby town or city. If the season or weather demands, find something to do indoors that will bring you joy, create memories, and take your mind off the tough stuff for a while.

Self-Care Tip: It is important to connect with others who have been where you are. Make connections through social media, a community-based support group, or your child's school district when they host informal meetings about special education. Life without a network can be lonely, so find your people.

7

Communicate with Teachers and School Staff

One of the most important relationships you can cultivate is with your child's elementary school teachers. Not only are their teachers providing your child's education, but they are also operating *in loco parentis* during the school day, in charge of your child's well-being when they're away from you. This chapter will explore ways to cultivate and maintain strong relationships with your child's teachers, service providers, and other school staff.

I've taught classes ranging from 18 to 32 children. I did as much as possible to interact with every child's parent. Even as an admitted workaholic, I had trouble staying in touch with every child's parent when my roster bulged with children. I always appreciated it when a parent reached out to me to ask about their child or to share a concern, as it helped me build a stronger relationship with them.

> **TIP** Your child's case manager plays a crucial role. This person oversees your child's IEP to ensure it's being followed. Sometimes, a child doesn't see their case manager daily. If that's the case, you'll want to establish communication norms with your child's case manager just as you would with their classroom teacher.

OPEN THE DIALOGUE

Many schools offer opportunities for kids to meet the teacher before the school year begins. Sometimes children can get into the school building, while other times these meet and greets are held in a centralized location. Attend those socials if your schedule permits since this is a low-pressure way to greet your child's teacher and express enthusiasm about working with them in the upcoming school year. If your child is anxious about the upcoming school year, you might go a little further.

Does Your Child Have Anxiety about School?

If so, contact your child's principal or special education supervisor to see if you can arrange a private meet and greet with their teacher during teachers' contracted back-to-school work days. Typically, teachers receive blocks of time to prepare their classrooms. For some kids, chatting with an unfamiliar adult is challenging. You could ask if your child can help the teacher organize the classroom library or math manipulatives for 15 minutes while you drop in to say hello. Helping out can break the ice between teacher and student.

It's important to begin a dialogue respectfully with your child's teacher, showing that you seek a positive and constructive relationship. One mother whose daughter has disabilities wrote the following letter to signal her desire to form a partnership and collaborate with the teacher to create a supportive learning environment for her child.

Dear Miss Hobart,

I hope this email finds you well as we embark on a new school year. I am writing to express my eagerness to collaborate with you for my child, Victoria "Vic" Bennett, who will be in your class this year.

Victoria has been recently diagnosed with autism and ADHD, and I believe that open and proactive communication between us will be key to supporting her success in the classroom. I would like to establish a partnership that allows us to stay connected regarding Vic's global progress, any challenges she may encounter, and strategies that enhance her learning experience.

I am open to discussing your most convenient communication channels, whether through email, scheduled meetings, or any other method that suits your preferences.

Additionally, if there are any specific accommodations or information you require regarding Vic's needs, please feel free to let me know, and I will provide you with that information.

Your expertise plays a crucial role in Vic's education, and I believe that working together will contribute to a positive and supportive learning environment. I appreciate your dedication to fostering an inclusive classroom, and I am confident that our collaboration will benefit Vic throughout the school year.

Thank you for your time and commitment to your students. I look forward to meeting and to a successful partnership and a fantastic school year!

Best regards,
Audra Bennett

Audra has had success using a version of this letter annually. She included the following information sheet as an attachment to her email to her daughter's teacher:

Meet Victoria "Vic" Bennett

★Takes medication at home daily; side effects include: increased hunger/thirst

Likes:

- Princesses
- Creating with LEGO
- Pretend play with costumes
- Helping with jobs
- Making friends/being silly
- Having a schedule
- Reading books
- Math

Challenges:

- Loud/overstimulating environments
- Abrupt changes in schedules
- Verbalizing wants or needs effectively

What works well:

- Having a daily visual schedule to track her progress
- Being prepped for big changes
- Verbal praise/encouragement
- Offering choices and breaks when applicable
- Having short- and long-term goals written and within view

Characteristics:

- Anxiety/Stress—fight or flight mode activation; hiding eyes/ reduced eye contact or difficulty verbalizing thought processes.
- Perseverations—asking/requesting/telling repeatedly within a short time frame.
  - **Vic may frequently ask about time or time left, over and over, when feeling stressed or anxious.**
- Flexibility—prefers control; has difficulty accepting "no." Uses coaching prompts via therapist to guide through inflexible moments:
  - Example: Asking a peer to play:
    - Vic: "Can I play with Jamie?"
    - Listener: "You can ask Jamie if he would like to play. If he says *'no,'* **how will you handle that**?"
    - Vic: I will answer "OK" and ask someone else.

A blank form that you can use—adapt it for your own child—is on page 118 and is also available to download at *www.guilford.com/shubitz-materials*.

Things You Need to Know About _____

Name:

Medications/Allergies:

Likes:

Dislikes:

What Works Well:

Characteristics:

Once a teacher responds, Audra asks further questions about the teacher's access and availability. For instance, what parameters should there be if the teacher prefers phone calls or texting? She asks if reaching out at night or on weekends is okay. Audra reconfirms whatever access the teacher has stipulated in an email so there's documentation. However, the bottom line is that she wants to build a relationship with her child's teacher in a way that works for the teacher's schedule. In addition, Audra asks for a short, informal meeting at the beginning of the school year so she can meet the teacher and find out how the beginning of Vic's school year is going.

> **TIP** Consider accepting a home visit. One of the schools I taught in asked teachers to step out of the school and into family homes. At first, I felt nervous walking into someone's home to meet them. After completing my first home visit, however, I realized the family was just as nervous as I was!
>
> I walked into those homes as a guest. I wasn't there to judge or snoop around. I was there to get to know the child and their family before the school year began.
>
> *Please consider opening your home to your child's teacher if they call and offer to do a home visit. It is a beautiful way to build rapport.*

SHARING INFORMATION AND CONCERNS

As a classroom teacher, I initiated most phone conversations with parents, usually regarding concerning behavior or incomplete work. Most parents didn't want to bother me unless their concern was urgent. But I didn't want parents to wait until their child had been tormented by another student at recess multiple times because they didn't want to bother me. I wanted to know *before* a situation escalated. I always said, *please reach out to me before a situation grows legs.* I encourage you to do the same with your child's teacher (or whatever staff member is closest to the issue) when your child tells you about something concerning that you don't feel you can manage alone. Here are some examples of when you might reach out:

- **Academic concerns:** Your child comes home feeling overwhelmed by the educational content, frustrated due to a challenging assessment, upset about a low score on a test, or unable to keep up with the academic demands of a subject area.

- **Behavioral concerns:** If you find out from your child or a teacher that your child received a consequence for their behavior, be prepared to inquire about it. It's essential to reach out if your child doesn't understand why they got in trouble or feels they were unjustly accused of something another child did (or participated in).

- **Family dynamics:** It's helpful to your child's teacher if they know when any aspect of your home life that you feel comfortable sharing is in flux—stress due to a job loss, surgery, diagnosis, or death of a loved one, for example.

- **Medication issues:** If you cannot access your child's regular medication or your child might need medical attention during a school day, please notify the teacher.

- **Participation and engagement:** Your child might share information that makes you wonder if and how much they're integrating into their classroom community. The only way to find out is to get details by asking questions.

- **Social-emotional well-being:** Everyone has a bad day. A major shift in your child's mood, sadness, persistent worry, or anxiety about social situations is worth bringing to the teacher's attention.

It helps to share your concerns anecdotally by sharing details as explained by your child without passing judgment. Reporting what you know as an informal and impartial narrative about your child's behavior, learning, or development helps keep correspondence brief while leaving room for the teacher to provide further insight into the situation. In addition, you can ask questions to help you clarify and better understand what's happening during the school day. I'll never forget the mother of one of my students, who epitomized the parent-teacher partnership and made me feel supported early in my career. Despite working two jobs, she always took the time to send in handwritten notes when needed, responded promptly when I reported a problem with her child's behavior, and with those simple measures made me feel even more eager to do well by her child.

Working as partners gives both parents and teachers opportunities to benefit the student. You must be on the same page because you're the people who spend the most time with your child right now. It helps to discuss potential solutions or informal accommodations when situations don't require an official IEP meeting. Once a consensus is reached about the next steps, responsibilities can be allocated to help solve the problem with support at school and home.

MAINTAIN AN ONGOING COMMUNICATION LOOP

It helps to schedule regular check-ins with your child's teacher via email, in person, or by phone. While most teachers will be willing to provide this to parents, as long as the frequency is reasonable, most teachers will not have the time to fit in multiple weekly in-person or phone check-ins with parents.

Using the method your child's teacher prefers, you might reach out about the following throughout the school year:

- Send information proactively: Let your child's teacher know if your child is facing an obstacle, a home life update, or a triggering event.
- Reinforcement: Tell the teacher if you're having trouble getting your child to read, practice math facts, or apply executive functioning strategies to their home life.
- Accommodations: Ask how the accommodations are used in the classroom and whether they benefit your child. Inquire about the skills they're gaining from their existing accommodations.
- Gratitude: Provide feedback to the teacher when things are going well. This helps teachers feel like they're benefiting your child.

So, where does that leave you if your child has greater support needs that you want to be aware of?

CHECK-IN/CHECK-OUT SHEETS

Many teachers use Check-In/Check-Out, or CICO, sheets (see Chapter 1) to help students with problematic or disruptive behaviors. CICO sheets are a Tier 2 PBIS intervention to help students meet behavioral goals. (This means every kid does *not* need a CICO sheet!) They provide students with genuine opportunities to talk with their teachers, self-reflect, and receive positive adult communication at school. The sheets vary from school to school, but I've provided two examples you can propose to your child's teacher, case manager, or IEP team to help your child during the school day. The sheets shown here are for upper elementary school students, but some teachers might use simpler forms for students in the primary grades.

The communication form shown on page 122, which I've adapted slightly, was created by Kyle Vercammen and Pamela Phillips for use with upper elementary school students.

Check-in/Check-out Log

Morning Check-in		
Date:	Morning Mindfulness: Close your eyes. Count your breaths to 10—in through the nose, out through the mouth. Count in your head: 1 for the in breath, 2 for the out breath, 3 in, 4 out…	
Use a feeling word to describe what you're feeling: (Pick a word on the feelings wheel)	Name one thing you are grateful for:	Name something you're proud of or something you love about yourself:
Calming Strategies: - Name your feelings - Ask for a break or help - Get a drink	- Write or draw - Tense and release your fists - Take a walk with an adult - Take deep breaths	- Give yourself an ear massage - Close your eyes and imagine a peaceful place - Positive self-talk

Daily Reflection					
GOALS	If I had a complaint about someone, I used a conflict resolution strategy to solve the issue.	If I had a question or didn't fully understand something, I asked for help from a peer or teacher.	If I feel like I failed or got something incorrect, I asked for feedback to better understand my error.	I was a leader of kindness today.	
My Observation	1 2 3 4 5	1 2 3 4 5	1 2 3 4 5	1 2 3 4 5	
Teacher Observation	1 2 3 4 5	1 2 3 4 5	1 2 3 4 5	1 2 3 4 5	
Comments					

Rubric

1 = I didn't meet my goal today.

2 = I did this a little bit, but less than half of the time.

3 = I did this about half the time, today.

4 = I met this goal most of the time!

5 = I completely met this goal today! Time to celebrate.

Rewards:

20-16 = Screen time and all other options.

15-14 = All options except screen time.

13 and below = Stay in class.

Reflection:

- Is your homework recorded? Y / N

- If you scored a 5 today, let's celebrate! High-five? Positive words? Teacher dance? Etc…

- If you scored a 3 or below, do you have strategies, tools, or ideas that could help you succeed next time? Y / N

If so, what are they?

If not, let's brainstorm:

Answer One or More:
How were you a leader today?
How were you kind today?
What's one thing you learned today?
What is one good thing that happened at school today?

Ben Wilson created the communication form below, which has been slightly adapted and was also created for upper elementary school students who change classrooms throughout the day.

Classroom Behavior Evaluation

Name: Date:

(Mark 0, 1, or 2. 2 means being successful and 0 needing work.)

Behavior	Science	Writing	Specials	Related Arts	Math	Reading	S.S.
Safe: Hands and body to self							
On-task: –Bring materials for class –Complete class work							
Accountable: On time for class							
Respectful: Respectful towards teachers and students Teacher initials							
Total points for the class							

Comments:

Adapted with permission from Ben Wilson.

The idea is for the teacher to fill it out with the student present so they can confer and offer words of affirmation for what is going well at the end of each period. A screenshot of the CICO sheet is sent home to the parent at the end of the school day.

An adaptation of Ben Wilson's form that has been filled in appears below.

Name: **Sue**   Date: **1/6/25**   Advanced Flight Plan:

(Mark 0, 1, or 2 with 2 being successful and 0 needs work)

Behavior	1st	2nd	3rd	4th	5th	6th	7th	
Safe: • Stay in designated area • Keep hands, feet, objects to self	②1 0	2̸ 1 0	②1 0	2̸ 1 0	②1 0	②1 0	2 1 0	
On-task: • Listen for instructions • Follow directions the first time • Be actively engaged	2①0	2②0	2①0	2̸ 0	2 1 ⓪	2①0	2 1 0	→ Got active with her group!
Accountable: • On time • Prepared to learn • Turn work in on time	2①0	2②0	2①0	2̸0	2①0	2①0	2 1 0	
Respectful: • Use professional language • Treat others kindly • Use materials for intended purposes	②1 0	②1 0	②1 0	2̸1 0	2①0	2①0	2 1 0	
Social Interaction • Interacts with peers	②1 0	2①0	②1 0	2̸1 0	2 1⓪	2①0	2 1 0	
Emotional Regulation • Ability to express and cope with emotions. • Positive Affect	②1 0	2①0	②1 0	2̸1 0	2 1⓪ *Slept*	2①0	2 1 0	
Teacher initials	JH	(e⊗	BTM	A	KM	CT	HZ	
Total points for the class	10	8	10	10	4	7	11	

Parent contact: ✓ (check if contact was made)   Total: / 56

↓ Very tired today

Ben Wilson form adapted and filled out by Betsy Hubbard with his permission and used here with permission from Betsy Hubbard.

CICO sheets are typically used in school to monitor a child's behavior. However, if a teacher snaps a photo of one and shares it via email, text, or a learning management system, it can also be a communication tool with parents. Keep in mind that they're a scaffold to improve a child's behavior, so they cannot be the sole way you learn about your child's school day.

COMMUNICATING THROUGH A LEARNING MANAGEMENT SYSTEM

Some teachers prefer to use the school's learning management system, or LMS, for electronic communications with parents since they have the system in front of them during the school day. Unlike email, communication with your child's teacher(s) through the LMS is usually deleted at the end of each school year. This isn't a big deal for run-of-the-mill communication. However, for substantial issues, you'll want to take screenshots or download communications to access them after the school year.

COMMUNICATING WITH RELATED SERVICE PROVIDERS

To play an important role in your child's growth, you ideally need to engage with everyone who interacts with your child. As you read in Chapter 3, many related service providers might work with your child depending on their disability and support needs. While a speech therapist will provide a progress report on a child's IEP goal(s), the van driver who transports a child to and from school will not. If your child has high support needs, keeping a list of who works with your child and how to contact them is essential. I suggest requesting a list of the people who work with your child from their case manager. Then you can create a master list on your phone or on paper. An example of how to set it up is on page 126 and is available to download at *www.guilford.com/shubitz-materials*.

_____ 's Service Providers

Name	Job Title	Contact Details	Preferred Contact Method	Frequency

Many related service providers have a lot of students on their caseload across multiple grades—and sometimes across multiple school buildings! I suggest establishing a preferred contact mode with these folks early in the school year if your child already has an IEP so you can easily reach them if you have a question, concern, or just want a general update.

NAVIGATE ISSUES

Jake is the father of three children, one of whom, Dakota, is neurodivergent and has a history of depression and anxiety, which is controlled with medication. Jake is a reporter who covers education for a newspaper. He manages all communication with Dakota's teachers. Over the years, he has learned not to be afraid to ask questions when unsure why something is happening or when Dakota tells him something that doesn't feel right.

One afternoon, Jake returned home to find Dakota distressed. Jake's in-laws had been watching the kids and reported that Dakota had been interrupting his sisters all afternoon, groaning whenever he wanted their attention, and stomping his feet whenever one of them spoke with one of Dakota's sisters. Once Jake's daughters were engaged in instrument practice and homework, Jake sat beside Dakota to determine what was wrong.

Eight-year-old Dakota cried and said the teacher had told him, "If you can't stop moving and bothering the people near you, you'll have to sit over there," meaning at a new desk on the perimeter of the classroom, where only one other kid sits. While physical breaks and flexible seating are part of Dakota's IEP, Jake felt frustrated that Dakota was moved away from his peers instead of being allowed to take a movement break outside the classroom.

As much as Jake wanted to send an angry email to Dakota's teacher, he knew he would be more likely to have a positive outcome for Dakota if his first email was not accusatory. He also knew that kids aren't always accurate about what's happening, so he started his email with, "Dakota said he . . . Is that right?"

Life is better for you and your child when you have a positive relationship with all the school personnel you deal with. However, things won't always go well. The question is, how will you manage it?

When a child comes home activated, sullen, or in hysterics, it's important to identify the problem. Parents usually get to the heart of the issue quicker when children have been provided appropriate communication tools so that they can help their parents understand what's troubling them and when they are also willing to discuss the issue. Once you assess the situation, contact the relevant school personnel or take no action.

I often ask my kids the following before determining my next steps:

- How can I help you?
- Is this a big deal or a small deal?
- Do you need my help to solve this problem, or can you sort this out tomorrow?
- Do you have the language you need to fix this independently, or would you like help practicing what you will say?

Once I ask these questions, I determine whether the issue needs to be conveyed to a teacher, service provider, or administrator. Anytime the issue involves a problem with another student or a grievance my child has with an adult, I ask my children to retell the situation calmly once they are more regulated. (Typically, I give them a snack and then discuss it.) As they talk, I take notes. Once I jot everything down, I ask them if they're telling me the whole truth or if there's anything they've exaggerated. I allow them to revise or edit their tale so I get a more nuanced idea of what happened. Then I craft an email. (See the conversation starters I often use in the box on page 128.) Before I send it, I ask my child to reread what I wrote, and have them correct any factual errors. I remind them that I want to contact the school only if they tell me the full truth. I promise them I won't be angry if they amend some of the details before I send the email. I do this because my children must understand that you don't complain whenever something bothers you. Once I read through the message again, I send it, and we carry on with our day.

You may think this is over the top. But let me tell you, I never want to accuse someone—a child or an educator—of a transgression because my child exaggerated or made up a story. I deeply respect educators and children. *My kids must understand I don't want to "use up my parental capital" by contacting someone at the school for minutiae or problems they can solve independently.* I've never regretted contacting the school after vetting my child's story.

> **TIP** Approach your child's teachers and all school community members with curiosity. People are less defensive when they're approached from a place of curiosity (not to be confused with passive-aggression) rather than in an accusatory manner. This will help you gather as much information as possible. If you discover from a teacher or school staff member that your child's IEP is not correctly implemented, it's time to advocate more strongly for your child's rights. Unless you or another trusted adult has observed something, initiate communication that leads with curiosity.

Email or Text Starters That Reflect Curiosity or Wondering

- My child told me [something]. Does that sound correct?
- I know kids often have a different impression than we do as adults ... so I wanted to check with you about [something] my child told me.
- Can you shed some light on [something] my child told me?
- My child mentioned [something]. Can you provide some insight into this?
- I wanted to follow up on my child's comment about [topic]. Can you tell me more about that?

Jake found out from the teacher's reply that Dakota had accurately reported what happened, but Jake learned more from Dakota's teacher about what caused him to be moved to the classroom's perimeter. Dakota's teacher explained that he had been rocking back and forth on the wiggle seat at his table, which meant he had bumped into the kids sitting beside him several times. Dakota's movement invaded other kids' personal spaces, which annoyed his tablemates. During group work, one of the kids stepped into Dakota's personal space, which caused him to yell at that child. To keep the peace, Dakota's teacher moved him away from his peers—to a desk on the perimeter of the classroom.

The teacher was frustrated and wanted the class controlled. However, Jake thought there were other ways to achieve this than marginalizing Dakota by sequestering him from his peers to work independently, which seemed like a punishment for having ADHD. As a result, Jake requested an IEP meeting. In the interim, he asked that Dakota receive break-request cards so he could take a break when needed to help him regulate his body and avoid invading other children's spaces. In addition, he asked that his son be reintegrated with his peers so he didn't feel ostracized.

ADDRESS PERSISTENT ISSUES

I'm the kind of parent who asks teachers to call me by my first name from day one. I do this to emphasize a team mentality and because I want them to view me as approachable. If I'm concerned about an issue happening with one of my kids, I bring it up to the teacher in a respectful way *without* cc'ing an administrator. There's no reason to escalate things when you can work on them respectfully and maturely. Sometimes teachers don't seem to change their approach despite multiple parent contacts. Yet I've been known to try to solve issues parent to teacher without administrator involvement.

A handful of times in my children's school careers, I have asked an administrator to intervene. Once I waited until early May to bring concerns to an administrator because I thought I could handle the situation. (Truth? The stress of the situation made me feel like my insides were being ripped apart.) Once I finished recounting what had happened, the administrator stated, "This is serious. Why did you wait so long to contact me?"

I felt sheepish. I didn't know what to say other than "I tried to solve this adult to adult."

That's when I learned that sometimes I have to escalate things since not all grown-ups adult in the same way. That experience taught me to take the following steps in the future:

1. Monitor ongoing problems. If something is unresolved after three contacts, contact the case manager, appropriate IEP team members, or administrator to request a meeting.
   o In an email, provide a *brief* overview of the issue since you don't want it to end up in a teacher's disciplinary folder. Save specifics for a phone call or in-person meeting.
2. Gather relevant data (such as behavior logs, data collection sheets, and written correspondence).
3. Communicate the issue or problem clearly. If you cannot propose solutions, ensure you'll work with the necessary people to resolve the issue.
4. Work collaboratively to solve the issue.
5. Make adjustments to your child's IEP if necessary.

A week later, Jake met with Dakota's IEP team to request additional support to help Dakota so he could get the movement he needed. The school's occupational therapist was already a consulting member of the IEP team. She lobbied to build structured sensory breaks into Dakota's daily schedule at a few key points during the school day. The IEP team brainstormed a short list of possible sensory breaks—doing rocket jumps and wall push-ups in the hallway, taking a short walk around the school, and jumping on a small trampoline—for Dakota. It took a few days, but ultimately they pulled together a variety of staff, which included two paraeducators and even the principal, to pick Dakota up at his classroom for a short break. Having a proactive approach to sensory breaks would give Dakota opportunities to move around without being punished for having the wiggles. In addition, Dakota would continue to have two break-request cards per day to use when he felt necessary.

The IEP team brainstormed other possibilities for Dakota besides the wiggle seat, which caused him to bump into classmates who sat beside him. Dakota could stand during cooperative group work or request his group move to the classroom meeting area where he could sit or lie prone while completing his work. While Dakota's teacher initially met varied seating options with some resistance, she agreed to try this.

Finally, Jake requested some classroom conversations about the differences in movement needs so classmates would understand why Dakota was doing what he was doing. Jake wanted the students to know that Dakota needed more activity and movement than most of his peers. The IEP team agreed to have Dakota's teacher work with the guidance counselor to initiate a classroom conversation about differing needs by opening a conversation with picture books that had neurodivergent main characters.

DEAL WITH THE PROBLEM OF MISSING PERSONNEL

I've heard about substitute teacher shortages for as long as I can remember. Then Covid came, and many educators retired from the profession. While a new crop of teachers is trained annually, there are staff shortages in most school districts. The problem is even more persistent in special education, where some special educators have left due to stressful working conditions, high caseloads, and a lack of resources to help them do their jobs well. Staff shortages can lead to inexperienced people being hired to fill in for trained instructional assistants and one-to-one aides (See Resources.). The special education shortages are a significant challenge that must be addressed.

Given these persistent staff shortages, especially in special education, it's understandable for parents to feel frustrated or powerless. However, there are steps you can take to advocate for your child despite these systemic issues. So, what can one parent do about a systemic problem? The only answer I can think of is to use your voice. Start with your child's case manager to ask what's happening. If the case manager, who is there to ensure your child's IEP is carried out, cannot help you, then request a face-to-face meeting with the building principal. Contact your LEA's special education director if you're unsatisfied with the response. If you cannot find a resolution to enable your child to get what they need *as outlined in their IEP,* you will have to escalate your concerns to a higher authority.

ESCALATE AS NEEDED

A challenging situation might require attention beyond your child's IEP team. In this case, the principal or special education director is important. When faced with difficulties and a lack of cooperation, addressing the issue through different channels and filing a formal complaint may be necessary. (See Chapter 3 for more details.) This filing creates an expectation that individuals involved will recognize the need for improvement and strive to make positive changes.

Before moving forward, contact a Community Parent Resource Center (CPRC), a Protection and Advocacy agency (P&A), or a Parent Training and Information Center (PTI), as defined in the Introduction. These organizations *should* be listed on the final page of your procedural safeguards book. Talking with other people can provide you with the next steps that could be helpful for your child.

REMEMBER TO COLLABORATE

Most teachers state that their most successful students with disabilities are the ones whose parents are collaborative. If the parents don't buy in, the child often doesn't do as well. They might be making progress but could progress more if there were collaboration between home and school.

Stay active in monitoring your child's progress and addressing challenges as they arise. You don't need to wait until something is wrong to reconvene the IEP team for a meeting. *You can call an IEP meeting anytime you need more people to tackle a problem your child is encountering at school.*

STAYING ON SOLID GROUND

Building a partnership with your child's teacher and service providers is essential to advocating for your child's education. Be the name they know. Ensure all relevant adults in your child's school know who your kid is. School personnel may roll their eyes when you call or see your name in their inbox, but you want them to take your call or reply to your email. You can establish a foundation for open communication and collaboration from day one. Keep in mind that your child's teachers work hard at their profession and are dedicated to educating each child in their classroom. And just like you, they have personal lives with commitments, families, and hobbies. They often cannot devote the time they would like to communicating with parents.

Remember, students thrive when parents and educators work together.

Tip for Cultivating Joy: Get involved with your child's school so the faculty, staff, and kids know who you are. Depending on your available time, some possibilities include running a special event for the parent-teacher organization, being a room parent, chaperoning class trips, and assisting with clerical work. Not only will this help you cultivate stronger relationships with the adults at your child's school, but you'll also be helping others by volunteering your time, which tends to bring people joy.

Self-Care Tip: A popular calming strategy is coloring. Scott M. Bea, PsyD, of the Cleveland Clinic, shares three reasons adult coloring can be calming: the attention flows away from ourselves, it relaxes the brain, and the low stakes make it pleasurable. Therefore, grab your colored pencils, crayons, or markers and an adult coloring book, and take some time to relax if you're feeling overwhelmed by whatever is happening with your child at school.

Part III

Embracing Opportunities

Making the Most of Nonschool Hours

8

Curate Joy

As the parent of a disabled child, you may find that worry has become your ever-present companion. At a time of great anxiety for me, I read an eye-opening book, *What You Wish For* by Katherine Center. On the surface, it's a romance novel. However, Center writes stories with emotional depth, humor, and hopeful themes. While *What You Wish For* deals with coping with a chronic medical condition and school shootings, Center balances out the serious stuff with essential messages about joy. One such message has stuck with me: "We made a choice to do joy on purpose. Not in spite of life's sorrows. But because of them."

After I closed Center's book, I knew I had to reclaim joy. I had no roadmap, but I learned more about joy from another book, *Joyful: The Surprising Power of Ordinary Things to Create Extraordinary Happiness* by Ingrid Fetell Lee. From Lee, I learned that joy isn't the same thing as happiness, but joy is a component of happiness. I started dressing in brighter colors. I played more games with my kids. I walked outside year-round. I made reading a novel before bedtime a habit. All of these things were in service of *doing joy on purpose.*

FINDING THE JOY THAT SURROUNDS US

I've built tips for cultivating joy into each chapter of this book because I now know how important it is to seek out joy actively. Lee has said it best: "We shouldn't put off joy until after we're out of a stressful situation. Instead, we should see joy as a tool for coping with stress. Joy is a form of resilience."

All parents must be resilient, especially when a child has higher support needs. We cannot take care of others if we are anguished. Besides self-care, actively seeking joy renews us and makes us happier. If we're more joyful, then joy has ripple effects on the people who matter most in our lives.

The tips for cultivating joy throughout the book have been for *you*. Now it's time to think about ways to seek joy *with and for your child!*

Before School

Unless you have kids who bounce out of bed—and *you* bounce out of bed as soon as your alarm goes off!—you know how gnarly mornings can get with children. Experiment with the following possibilities to see what makes you and your child more joyful.

Games

When my daughter was 11, she wanted in on the fun I was having with Wordle. Together, we solved the puzzle each morning, and she moved on to Spellie, similar to Wordle but for kids. After my son turned five, he also became interested. I began creating custom Wordle-like puzzles for him since the official ones were too challenging. Once Nell Duke, a professor of literacy, language, and culture at the University of Michigan, published "What Wordle Reminds Us About Effective Phonics and Spelling Instruction," I knew I was using screen time in not just a joyful way but a beneficial way too.

Over time we found other phone- and tablet-based games. Our interest levels have ebbed and flowed, but other favorites of ours that you might consider are:

- *The New York Times:* Connections, Spelling Bee, Strands, Tiles
- *The Washington Post:* Daily Mini Meta Crossword, Keyword, On the Record

Mindfulness

I meditate first thing in the morning. Meditation helps me be centered before I interact with my family. It creates a state of mindfulness, which I need first thing in the morning.

On weekdays, I set my phone down on the kitchen counter before I make breakfast. I tend to eat oatmeal daily. Therefore, there's a rhythm to making my breakfast. First, I take out the pot, measure water, and turn on the stove. While that heats to a boil, I remove the oats from the pantry and beverages and maple syrup from the refrigerator. I tend to do things in the same order so I don't miss a step before I'm caffeinated. Finally, I sit down at the table to eat breakfast with my son. If there's something he asks that requires Google or a phone app, it waits until after we eat. Cooking and eating without distractions brings me joy since it lets me focus entirely on my son while we eat breakfast.

In "The Power of Mindfulness," Juliann Garey explains mindfulness as a "[M]editation practice that begins with paying attention to breathing in order to focus on the here and now—not what might have been or what you're worried could be. The ultimate goal is to give you enough distance from disturbing thoughts and emotions to be able to observe them without immediately reacting to them." She explains how doing something as simple as teaching a child to pay attention to their breathing is a way to start a mindfulness practice.

The UMass Memorial Health Center for Mindfulness says that "Patients often report greater joy for the simple things in life, such as a shared moment with their child or partner or more aware of the change of seasons as flowers bloom and snow falls. We begin to realize that there is more 'right' with us than 'wrong' with us as we become more engaged in our lives." I couldn't agree more.

Find online resources for engaging your child in a mindfulness practice in the Resources at the back of the book.

Music

In the summer of 2024, my kids became *obsessed* with the overture of a singer's live concert album. It was wordless and, like most overtures, included shortened versions of the best songs on the album. "Do you think this overture would be good for me to play on the days the two of you won't get out of bed?" "Yes!" they responded enthusiastically. From then on, I started playing the overture on rainy mornings when one or both kids needed something uplifting to help them get out of bed.

In "How Listening to Music Can Have Psychological Benefits," Kendra Cherry explains 10 research-backed benefits of music. Listening to music benefits us in many ways, including improving cognition, memory, mood, motivation, and reducing stress.

Energetic music can boost our mood and increase joy and enthusiasm, whereas calming music can help us relax and unwind, leading to a more joyful state of mind. Consider creating a playlist of music you enjoy with your child to create a more joyful start to the day.

Reading

One of my most vivid memories of living in New York City is taking the subway to and from work in the summertime before the subways were air-conditioned. The misery of sweaty humans packed into each car at rush hour was palpable—except for those reading books or the newspaper. These folks always seemed content no matter whose skin was pressed against theirs. Why? Their minds were elsewhere, not focusing on the tightness and scent of urban existence.

Mornings with kids are hectic, especially if you have a child who relies on you for assistance with their ADL, which is occupational therapy's short-hand for activities of daily living. I am not suggesting you read a picture book while preparing breakfast or wrangling a child to brush their teeth properly. But how about reading a poem a day from an anthology? Most poems are short, can be read in less than a minute, and can be used as an entry point into a conversation with your child. If your kid likes to laugh, choose a book of humorous poems. If they want to learn about a specific topic, choose a book of poems rich in sensory detail. Select whatever brings you and your child joy!

Need a starting point? For the sake of space, I'll point you toward Lee Bennett Hopkins, one of the most outstanding children's poetry anthologists. Some of my favorite anthologies Hopkins compiled are *Days to Celebrate: A Full Year of Poetry, People, Holidays, History, Fascinating Facts, and More; I Remember: Poems and Pictures of Heritage, Nasty Bugs; Sharing the Seasons: A Book of Poems;* and *Wonderful Words: Poems About Reading, Writing, Speaking, and Listening.* Also, poet Amy Ludwig VanDerwater's The Poem Farm allows you to search for poems by topic. You'll find what you're looking for on the shelves of your local library or bookstore.

After School

Once the school day ends, it's time to shift gears and focus on play, extracur-ricular activities, family time, and wind-down time. But before we do, I must address the elephant in the room: homework.

"Is homework helpful or harmful?" It's a question a few of my Two Writing Teachers colleagues and I set out to answer in 2017. (See Resources.) It reflected our concerns about homework trends and our thinking based on research and study. The posts in that mini-series sought to help our audience of educators reimagine homework, think about underlying assumptions about homework, reinvent nightly writing assignments, and involve family members with writing at home.

Without a clear purpose, assigning homework to elementary school students doesn't have their best interests at heart. There is no clear proof that homework reinforces learning, improves achievement or study skills, or teaches responsibility. I believe the adverse effects of homework, which can include an impact on mental health, far outweigh the benefits of moderate homework.

Admittedly, I didn't know better when I began teaching in 2004. I assigned nightly homework, plus 40–50 minutes of reading. Nowadays, I am on a soapbox dedicated to eradicating homework in elementary school. Alfie Kohn, author of 14 books that focus on education and parenting, including *The Homework Myth,* wrote the following in 2012: "We parents need to reach out to others in our communities to debunk uninformed assumptions ('homework is academically beneficial'), to challenge silly claims ('homework is needed to provide a link between school and family'), and to help restore sanity and joy to our children's lives."

Your child shouldn't come home after seven hours to do more work! There are plenty of other things kids can do that will bring them joy during the second shift of their day.

Homework Alternatives

Reading every night instead of doing homework *is* proven to help kids. As a certified literacy specialist and someone who believes kids should have a say in what they read, I believe that children should engage in self-selected reading at home daily. Most kids' school days are spent reading materials selected by others, so they need the choice to read something they understand and enjoy at home. As educator Donalyn Miller states, "When we diminish a child's reading choices, we diminish the child."

Reading *to* and *alongside* children is highly beneficial. (We'll discuss this further in the next chapter.)

Kids should be passionate about the assignments they're creating at home. For instance, in a 2022 article, reporter Sarah Wood quotes Harris Cooper, author and professor emeritus of psychology and neuroscience at Duke

University, "Assignments can be fun, like having students visit educational locations, keep statistics on their favorite sports teams, read for pleasure or even help their parents grocery shop. The point is to show students that activities done outside of school can relate to subjects learned in the classroom."

An Alternative to Traditional Homework: Google employees are provided with personal development time, which makes up one-fifth of their workweek. The 20% time rule allows Google employees to learn new skills or pursue interests. The 20% time rule leads to innovation and sparks creativity. What if schools took a cue from Google? Perhaps if kids were allowed to pursue something of interest after-school hours, it could lead to greater fulfillment, academic success, and joy!

Play

The United Nations Convention on the Rights of the Child is a human rights treaty that outlines the specific rights of children and sets standards for their protection and well-being. It was adopted by the United Nations General Assembly in 1989 and ratified by almost all countries worldwide. The 31st of the 54 articles deals with the importance of play, which is fundamental to children's development and well-being. It states that the parties to the treaty:

1. . . . recognize the right of the child to rest and leisure, to engage in play and recreational activities appropriate to the age of the child and to participate freely in cultural life and the arts.
2. . . . shall respect and promote the right of the child to participate fully in cultural and artistic life and shall encourage the provision of appropriate and equal opportunities for cultural, artistic, recreational, and leisure activity.

Playing is a basic human right of all children. Through research and play advocates, we know that play is a natural way to learn and the "work" of childhood. Play can involve decision making, interacting, laughing, problem solving, and smiling. It supports imagination, self-determination, and diminished self-consciousness. Yet many kids who have disabilities spend after-school hours at medical or therapy appointments or working with tutors. Without even realizing it, many parents—in an effort not to have their kids miss school—inadvertently swap after-school playtime with these necessary appointments. This is unfortunate.

Pam Muñoz Ryan, an award-winning children's author, has spoken publicly about the beauty of her "unchoreographed childhood" resulting from her parents' "benevolent neglect." This concept highlights the value of unstructured time for children, allowing them to learn how to occupy themselves and work through boredom. However, remember that most children thrive on routine, so unstructured time may have to be left for weekends, as discussed on page 145. Another reality to consider is all the after-school activities available for children to enroll in. It's tempting for parents to try to pack every hour after school with something. So you may have to model how to allow some empty spaces in their day by also allowing some in yours. Research shows that many adults, especially parents, feel too busy to enjoy life. You can combat this by prioritizing activities that bring joy to all of you and avoid unnecessary commitments—yours and for your children's.

> **TIP** Provide a list of screen-free options for this "unchoreographed time" and model how to use them productively.

We bond with our children when we play with them. If you want to increase your joy and build more play into your daily life as a parent, The LEGO Foundation's online resources are a fantastic place to begin. (See Resources.)

Dinnertime

Ever since our children's sleep schedules have been in sync, we've prioritized family dinners. The time we sit down together fluctuates based on everyone's schedules. Usually, this means eating early or later than the ideal 6:00 p.m. Even though the chef (me!) hears complaints about something being too spicy or not being the vegetable they wanted, I relish the four of us sitting together. It's a chance to catch up on the day, reflect, and plan for the future. Through the years, I've found a few ideas to make family dinner conversation less mundane.

Silliest Part of the Day

Life can be filled with annoyances, but looking at those everyday moments and noting something silly that happened can get everyone giggling and add a tiny bit of joy. It takes a few days to get this idea up and running, but focusing on the most ridiculous part of the day forces us to reframe what may have been initially frustrating and allows us to find the humor in it. (See Resources.)

Three Good Things

I've adopted the practice of having each family member write down three good things and then ask everyone to share them. The "good things" don't have to be about that day; they are positive things that happened during the week. You can invite younger children to tell you their three good things and have you write them down, or they can draw a picture of them and share their picture. Regardless, having an authentic gratitude practice helps us feel more joyful. (See Resources.)

After-School Activities of Any Kind

Young children need exposure to many different activities to determine their interests. While helping kids discover their interests and passions is helpful, it usually means investing money and time (including shuttling them there and back). Unless you have a lot of both, picking and choosing after-school activities that align with your child's interests, schedule, and budget is crucial.

- Money: Many public school districts, municipalities, and local community centers offer lower-cost activities to residents. Start looking at your township or county's parks and recreation department newsletter or website to see if affordable options match your child's interests and schedule.

- Time: Think about the time it takes to shuttle your child back and forth to activities. Then factor in the time you'll spend sitting on a field or in a waiting room for them. Is the time investment worth it? Does your child derive joy from the activity? If the answer to both questions is yes, keep doing what you're doing!

Parents who work until 5:00 or 6:00 P.M. and pick their child up from an after-school program are faced with the dilemma of what to do afterward. Do you take them to Cub Scouts or a music lesson, or go home, eat dinner, and relax? I know this may be an unpopular opinion, but keep it simple. It's okay to limit your kiddo to one activity on weeknights that brings them joy, so you aren't shuttling them around town after you finish your workday. (With two kids, I limit my kids to one weeknight activity and one weekend activity.) That's exhausting. They need to rest—and so do you!

Know When to Say "Uncle"

My daughter had been in ballet and tap for over a year when she decided she hated wearing tights. After struggling to get her into tights, I realized she might not enjoy dance anymore or was too tired after kindergarten. Instead of forcing her, I let her quit at the end of the month and withdrew her from the dance school. We then enrolled her in a visual arts class and an aerial arts class, which suited her better.

Weekends

When children were asked whether they felt positive about the future in one survey, about two-thirds of those who engaged in fun activities with their families had a more positive outlook on the future, whereas 41% of children who don't do fun things with their families felt less optimistic about their future. Shared family time is important. But most parents work, and most kids have a fairly packed schedule during the week. So weekends—or whatever days of the week you all have off together—are the time to try to share joy. Here are a few ideas.

Adventures and Exploration Close to Home

My favorite weekend activities with my family include walking on rail trails and hiking in parks. But it's important to cater to your child's interests. Even though I like hiking, one of my kids doesn't. So, I try to attach hikes to something pleasurable (like going out for ice cream) at the end of the hike. I also recommend spending one-on-one time with each of your kids if you have two or more and have reliable childcare.

For new ideas, I check the websites of my local library and the township's parks and recreation department to see what's happening. They compile lists of local events that allow us to try new things while staying close to home.

In addition, I often check these sites to help me find novel things to do with my family at low or no cost:

- **AllEvents** has an app and a website dedicated to helping you find events in any area. Simply input your location, select kids, state whether you want the events to be free or paid, and see what's coming up in your area.

- **Clipp** provides coupons and deals for restaurants, stores, museums, and other activities (such as bowling and mini golf) in your vicinity.

- **Groupon** offers deals for families on local attractions, making amusement parks, movies, and youth sports more affordable.

- **Mommy Poppins** is an online guide that provides listings for activities in major cities and a roundup of ideas that answer the question "What should I do today?"

- **Tripadvisor** is my go-to place for honest travel reviews. Their site has a "things to do" function, which allows you to type in an activity, attraction, destination, or place. The search feature will then provide you with ideas.

Family Game and Movie Nights

For movie nights at our house, we pop a couple of popcorn bags, pass out cozy blankets, and watch together. As for game nights, we gather around the table and pick a game. My children's favorite is Monopoly, but that gets competitive. When both were younger, we mixed in games from Peaceable Kingdom, which creates cooperative group games that allow children to play well together. Both game and movie nights are a fantastic way to bond as a family without the added expense and fuss of going out. If your kids have different interests and are relatively far apart in age, let them take turns choosing the movie or the game.

Community Service

Bring joy to yourself while making the world a better place for others by volunteering your time as a family. Many food banks and soup kitchens do not allow elementary school children to volunteer. Therefore, if your school or house of worship doesn't provide volunteer opportunities, here is a list of things you can do *with* your child:

- Take a meal to someone caring for a new baby or recovering from surgery.
- Clean up a local park.
- Collect and donate gently used books to a Little Free Library, local library, or school.
- Create cards and send them to a local nursing home, to veterans, or overseas troops.

- Make care packages of essential items for a local homeless shelter.
- Organize a food drive for a local food bank or animal shelter.
- Visit nursing homes.
- Volunteer at an animal shelter.
- Welcome new neighbors with baked goods.

Recently, a member of our religious congregation had surgery. I offered to make some meals for her. My kids helped make her dessert, and they colored pictures to cheer her up. They also accompanied me on the food delivery to wish her well. I realize we didn't create world peace, but bringing joy to someone else's corner of the world matters.

Watch a Sunset

In December 2022, my kindergartner son wanted to go to the top of the Empire State Building. Despite my reservations about the touristy visit and the cold, I paid the surcharge for sunset access when all daytime tickets were sold out. After exploring Midtown Manhattan for two hours, we reached the observatory at sunset. Watching the sun dip below the skyline was a profound experience and created a cherished memory for both of us.

Discuss eye safety related to the sun, then take time to watch a sunset with your child and embrace the experience together.

School Vacations during the Academic Year

Long weekends and week-long school breaks can be disruptive for children who thrive on routine and structure. While these breaks can wreak havoc on the day-to-day routines you create, they also offer extended opportunities for joy.

I interviewed many parents for this book and always asked where they find joy. One mother said:

> "You let the joy come to you. As a family, we love watching football. We go to one home NFL game per year. Spending time watching football has become a regular fixture in our lives. We travel to all-inclusive resorts, not large theme parks, since the crowds and noise are too much for my child. Our family looks forward to this vacation each year since we've found that all-inclusive places offer us less stress as parents since we can do as little or

as much as we want because everything is there. We may not go on big, splashy vacations overseas like other families, but we've created experiences that work for our family. We discovered that the annual football game and vacation week bring us joy."

Many families visit museums and attend performances during school breaks. Visiting a museum or attending a performance doesn't have to be expensive. Many museums and arts centers offer discounted or free admission one day per month. In addition, many museums offer reduced or free admission to individuals with disabilities and one of their caregivers.

Summer Vacation

The demands of having kids home for 10–12 weeks every summer can be exhausting. Add in medical and therapy appointments for your child with a disability or chronic health condition, and summertime is just stressful. When you're in the thick of things, working through a specific issue, it's hard to hit pause on therapy for more than a week. However, some therapists will suggest a therapy vacation for a month of summer since the longer pause can help kids integrate what they learned and apply it to their summertime lives. Believe it or not, a longer pause can be beneficial for kids! Talk with your child's providers to determine if and when your child is ready for a therapy pause.

Summer vacation offers extended opportunities for joy. Planning is the key! The Greater Good Science Center at the University of California, Berkeley, has compiled extensive resources to help parents plan for summer using five lenses: play, creativity, flow, games, and humor. (See Resources.) While not all of the articles and podcasts will be right for you, this resource list can be the catalyst to help you kickstart your summertime planning.

Another way to approach summer vacation is by creating a bucket list of ordinary things you can enjoy together. Once you complete a list of inside and outside things, you can work together to decide based on the weather and everyone's mood. If you're struggling to decide what to do, use a random decision maker to gamify what to do next.

Specialty Programs

Many service organizations, hospitals, and universities run summer programs for children with disabilities or chronic medical conditions. Check with your school district, regional education service agency, or PTI for a list of resources in your area.

iCan Shine runs three recreational activity programs—iCan Bike, iCan Swim, and iCan Dance—for children and young adults with disabilities. These five-day programs teach and empower people with disabilities to bike, swim, or dance with confidence. (The biking program is for people aged eight and over, while the swimming and dance programs are for those three and up.) iCan Shine partners with local organizations to host week-long camps at approximately 100 sites in 35 states and three provinces in Canada. The fee for iCan Shine depends on the location, but it ranges from $100 to $250.

Day Camps

Day camps encourage socialization, skill development, and recreation during the summer months. Accredited day camps provide parents with safe places to send their children with hours similar to the school day. Some day camps provide before and after care, which can help working parents who need more childcare coverage than the average day camp offers. Even with an extended day, most day camps are more affordable than overnight camps.

In some parts of the country, it's challenging to find traditional day camps that span eight weeks and offer various activities that expose campers to the arts, land sports, water sports, and nature. Sometimes camps offer only week-long (full- and half-day) thematic sessions. Examples are academic enrichment (such as STEM), adventure, arts and performance, nature, religion, scouting, specialty (like cooking or robotics), sports, and travel camps. Multiple week-long sessions allow families to dip in and out of camp as their summer schedule permits. In addition, they allow kids to have a breadth of summertime experiences. (See the box on page 150 for resources that assist with finding a camp.) Keep in mind, moving from camp to camp each week can be challenging for kids who struggle with new routines or meeting new people, so check in with your child before you reserve spots for them in different camps.

Many day camps believe in inclusion so that children with disabilities are grouped alongside nondisabled peers. When done with intention, inclusive day camp experiences benefit all campers.

There's another kind of camp, sometimes called "special needs camps." These camps serve children with disabilities, are run and staffed by trained professionals, and are well-staffed with trained counselors who provide greater support to the campers. Some camps offer behavioral/emotional support, while others are disability-specific, sensory-focused, or therapeutic. These camps can be an excellent fit for children who might thrive better with activities tailored to their disability or support needs while providing opportunities for independence and increased self-esteem in an environment with a lower staff-to-camper ratio. (These exist as sleepaway camps as well.)

Ways to Find a Camp

The American Camp Association has accredited over 20,000 traditional, specialty, and special needs camps across the United States. You can search their online database by session length, co-ed/single sex, specialty, or special needs. You can also do an internet search for "{disability/medical condition} + day camp for kids" to find day camps near you.

In addition, specialized companies work with parents to match their children with the best possible camp. Look for businesses that do not charge families directly. Typically, they receive a modest fee from camps for facilitating successful introductions or after your child attends the camp. (See Resources.)

Sleepaway Camps

Some children begin attending sleepaway camps when they're in upper elementary school. However, the idea of sending away a child with higher support needs to sleepaway camp can be, well, terrifying! It's essential to do a readiness assessment, which many sleepaway camps post on their website. Your child's age, interest level, and ability to successfully stay overnight with family or friends are three of the things that a readiness assessment measures.

Traditional Sleepaway Camps

Like day camps, many traditional sleepaway camps include kids with disabilities in the general community. Some traditional sleepaway camps will add a counselor to the bunk to decrease the counselor-to-camper ratio, providing more support to campers. At other camps, bunks may be for kids with similar learning, behavioral, or social profiles. While these children live together in a bunk with counselor support, they eat in the same dining hall and engage in the same activities as the rest of the camp population.

Before signing the camp contract, you can visit a camp to understand what it's like when their summer programming is underway. If that's not possible, speak with the director to see what kinds of accommodations and supports will be in place to help your child. Furthermore, request the names of returning campers' parents with needs similar to your child's. These conversations will provide a candid assessment of how the camp staff helped their child feel included. You want your child's time at overnight camp to be transformational, but you must interview a few camps to ensure you're picking the right one.

Specialized Overnight Camps

There are sleepaway camp options tailored to disabilities or medical conditions. Being with other kids who are similar to them—medically, socially, and behaviorally—is helpful. Children don't have to worry about fitting in in these situations because all other campers *get it*. As a result, sleepaway camps that are "therapeutic camps" or "medical specialty camps" provide kids with a break from being *different*.

Just as you might try a new medical therapy for your child, a specialized sleepaway camp is one of the best gifts you can give to your child. Having a chronic disease, neurodivergence, disability, or other impairments can take a toll on a child. Allowing your child to have a place where they belong that their siblings or classmates aren't a part of can benefit their self-esteem. Life can be successful and joyful at these sleepaway camps because the community understands, accepts, and supports them.

As parents, we cannot create this for our children at home. For many of us, sending our child to camp is out of our comfort zone. However, without parents at camp, children are often far more capable than teachers or parents allow at school or home. Joy is abundant when kids try new things at camp and experience success celebrated *with* their peers but *without* a parent or teacher.

Specialty overnight camps allow children to be with and find their people.

Summer Learning Loss

Summer learning loss refers to the decline in math, reading, and writing skills among elementary school students during the summertime. Most community-based and online resources for elementary school students are summer reading programs. I encourage you to explore what exists in your area.

Many think drill and practice apps, packets, and workbooks will help kids keep and refine their skills; these things are a joy-killer. Often, kids slog through summertime skill practice, which can diminish their engagement and desire to learn. Visit the online resources (*www.guilford.com/shubitz-materials*) for authentic ways to engage your child in literacy and math during the summer.

PLAYTIME, DOWNTIME, AND FAMILY TIME

Challenge Success is a nonprofit organization affiliated with Stanford University Graduate School of Education that focuses on academic achievement and mental health. They assert that every child needs daily playtime, downtime, and family time, or PDF, for healthy development. These things daily increase the child's and family's health and well-being. Their website defines each aspect of PDF and provides tip sheets for helping different age bands of kids, including children in elementary school, with a daily dose of PDF. (See Resources.) You'll find that the PDF Tips reflect the essence of this chapter. To increase joy, we must ensure our child has these things built into their lives.

You've probably noticed several references to my love of reading in this chapter. I believe reading, more specifically *stories,* can be infused into all three aspects of PDF. Come along with me to Chapter 9, where I'll show you how reading together is essential to building literacy skills, learning new things, and creating joyful experiences between a child and their parent.

Tip for Cultivating Joy: Watch filmmaker Louie Schwartzberg's TED Talk "Nature. Beauty. Gratitude." It will inspire you to pay greater attention to the natural world, the beauty of people, and the modern-day wonders surrounding you. Schwartzberg's inspiring talk will not only help you cultivate a gratitude practice, since one of the best tools we have to activate the best version of ourselves is gratitude. Also, this short TED Talk will help you think about ways to find joy every day you are gifted. (See Resources.)

Self-Care Tip: Learn about the benefits of self-compassionate touch. Research from Aljoscha Dreisoerner and Eli Susman has shown that soothing self-touch can lower cortisol levels and heart rate, thereby reducing stress. The effects of self-compassionate touch are dependent on cultivating a consistent daily practice. Learn more about making self-soothing touch a habit by listening to one or both of the following episodes of The Science of Happiness podcast. (See Resources.)

9

The Power of Reading Together

Over a decade ago, I needed a new author headshot, and the photographer agreed to include a family shoot afterward. It was a perfect May morning to take photos in a botanical garden. We took many posed photos, but my favorite one from that day was of my husband and me sitting with our daughter on a blanket while I read *Knuffle Bunny Too* by Mo Willems. It was one of her favorite books, so she looked delighted in the photos. Every time I look at that photo, I think about how my husband and I have bonded with our daughter over books. There are a bunch of books I hang on to—that both of my kids are "too old" for—simply because they bring a warm feeling to my chest since I read certain books repeatedly to my children.

Reading alongside your child has enormous benefits. Books in various genres allow children to delight in stories, learn new information, and be mesmerized by language.

One way children learn language is by hearing lots of books read aloud to them. A study by Jessica Logan of The Ohio State University found that children whose parents read them five books a day before the beginning of kindergarten had been exposed to approximately 1.4 million more words than children who weren't read to before kindergarten. (Some people refer to this as the "million-word gap.") The study found that reading one picture book daily to a child results in the child's hearing 78,000 words per year. While this won't add up to a million, it shows that a book a day can lead to positive outcomes. And, of course, parents talk to their child, which not only exposes them to but also helps them understand spoken language.

Even as a literacy specialist who knows the benefits of reading aloud, I am unsure if I read five books a day to each of my children daily for the first five years of their lives. Some days, I read them more than five books, especially when board books were part of their daily diet. But as the books became longer, I read fewer than five. My mother-in-law, a teacher and reading specialist, reminded me that my kids would be okay since they understood the Concepts of Print, which means children understand the features and behaviors that support reading acquisition. Therefore, if your child is unaware of some of these concepts, you can help them learn them by reading together regularly. All you have to do is model your thinking about how books go, and they'll begin to pick up on the concepts.

Many people think they stop reading aloud to their children in upper elementary school, when many kids can read and comprehend longer books independently. You can stop, but I encourage you to continue. The books you read might change because your kids may wish to read middle-grade novels instead of picture books. However, finding books you can read and enjoy together as part of a bedtime routine is a fabulous way to bond over books. Unless your child wishes to read aloud to you, this is a time for *you* to read aloud *to* your child. In doing this, you're not only reading a book you can discuss with your child but also modeling a love of reading. All kids need to see that, even sixth graders!

I'll never forget when my daughter, who was 10 at the time, asked me to read her *El Deafo* by Cece Bell at bedtime. I was unsure what to do since *El Deafo* is a graphic novel, a genre I was unfamiliar with. I called for help on my Facebook page, and many people gave me tips about how to read a graphic novel aloud to my child meaningfully. With their help, we got to experience a book of her choosing together.

Before we move further, I need to stand on my soapbox momentarily: *All reading counts. If your child is reading a graphic novel, they're reading! If your child wants to read an audiobook, they're reading! The same goes for magazines, ebooks, comic books, and technical materials. Reading is reading! No matter what your sister-in-law, neighbor, co-worker, or a stranger says, all forms of reading count as reading!*

INCLUSIVE READING EXPERIENCES

Children need to read books that affirm their disability experiences. In addition, all kids can benefit from books that teach them about disabilities they don't have. This can help a child to be an ally to disabled classmates, friends, and family members.

Rudine Sims Bishop, a renowned scholar of multicultural children's literature who is a professor emerita of education at The Ohio State University, is known for the concept of *books as mirrors, windows, or sliding glass doors*. She wrote:

> Books are sometimes windows, offering views of worlds that may be real or imagined, familiar or strange. These windows are also sliding glass doors, and readers have only to walk through in imagination to become part of whatever world has been created or recreated by the author. When lighting conditions are just right, however, a window can also be a mirror. Literature transforms human experience and reflects it back to us, and in that reflection we can see our own lives and experiences as part of the larger human experience. Reading, then, becomes a means of self-affirmation, and readers often seek their mirrors in books.

It is critically important for your child to have books that mirror their life experiences. Sometimes representation is a book that teaches about disability, while other times, there's a child who has a disability in the story, but that isn't the book's central message. It's just about a child with a disability living their life. Books like that matter, too! The bottom line is that *kids need mirrors, windows, and sliding glass doors to help them develop empathy and self-worth*.

OWN VOICES

Nondisabled writers have written some of the books below. Others are by Own Voices authors, writers who share identities with the characters they create.

Authors writing from lived experience add nuance, authenticity, and understanding that are difficult to replicate through research alone or from an outsider's viewpoint, no matter how astute and empathetic. Unfortunately, marginalized groups have often had their stories told by others, sometimes loaded with harmful representation and inaccuracies. As a parent, you play a crucial role in shaping your child's understanding of their disability and the world. Supporting authors who write from their own lived experiences is a valuable way to do this.

APPROACHES TO BUILDING A DIVERSE READING LIST

You'll notice that some parts of the list are more extensive than others. Certain types of disabilities have more books than I could even list, while there's a shortage of others. Take this as an opportunity. Perhaps it's time for you to tell your story!

In addition, some books could fit into more than one category. For instance, I put *Benji, the Bad Day, and Me* in the books for siblings category, but it deals with neurodiversity. Another example is *It's So Difficult,* which I placed in the mental health section, but also deals with sensory issues and communication. I put books about dyslexia in the learning disabilities section, but they could easily be classified under neurodivergence.

This list includes a handful of biographical picture books. However, it is by no means exhaustive. There are *many* more biographies out there that chronicle the lives of disabled people.

Unless otherwise noted, the majority of the list below comprises picture books (nonfiction and fiction) and early readers. There are a handful of middle-grade novels, novels in verse, and graphic novels on the list.

RECOMMENDED BOOKS

General

- *Fighting For Yes! The Story of Disability Rights Activist Judith Heumann* by Maryann Cocca-Leffler and Vivien Mildenberger (New York: Abrams, 2022)
- *Hazel's Best Day: A Story of Community, Accessibility, and Pride in Being Yourself* by Adiba Nelson and DeAnn Wiley (New York: Feiwel & Friends, 2026)
- *I Am Not a Label: 34 Disabled Artists, Thinkers, Athletes and Activists from Past and Present* by Cerrie Burnell and Lauren Baldo (London: Wide Eyed Editions, 2020)
- *Included: A Book for ALL Children About Inclusion, Diversity, Disability, Equality and Empathy* by Jayneen Sanders and Camila Carrossine (Macclesfield, Victoria, Australia: Educate2Empower, 2022)
- *This Is How We Play: A Celebration of Disability and Adaptation* by Jessica Slice, Caroline Cupp, and Kayla Harren (New York: Dial Books, 2024)
- *You Are Enough: A Book About Inclusion* by Margaret O'Hair and Sofia Cardoso, inspired by Sofia Sanchez (New York: Scholastic, 2021)

Books for Siblings

- *Benji, the Bad Day, and Me* by Sally J. Pla and Ken Min (New York: Lee & Low Books, 2018)

- *Me and My Sister* by Rose Robbins (Grand Rapids, MI: Eerdman Books for Young Readers, 2020)
- *Terrible Horses* by Raymond Antrobus and Ken Wilson-Max (Somerville, MA: Candlewick Press, 2024)

Books for Friends

- *I Can Help* by Reem Faruqi and Mikela Prevost (Grand Rapids: Eerdmans, 2021)
- *My Friend Has ADHD* by Amanda Doering Tourville and Kristin Sorra (Bloomington, MN: Picture Window Books, 2010)
- *Remarkable Remy* by Melanie Heyworth and Nathaniel Eckstrom (Richmond, VA: Bright Light, 2023)
- *Sensitive* by Sara Levine and Mehrdokht Amini (Minneapolis: Carolrhoda Books, 2023)
- *The Boy with Flowers in His Hair* by Jarvis (Somerville, MA: Candlewick Press, 2022)

Chronic Medical Conditions

- *Aniana Del Mar Jumps In* by Jasmine Mendez (New York: Dial Books, 2023)
- *Dancing in the Storm* by Amie Darnell Specht and Shannon Hitchcock (New York: Rocky Pond Books, 2024)
- *Featherless/Desplumado* by Juan Felipe Herrera and Ernesto Cuevas, Jr. (San Francisco: Children's Book Press, 2004)
- *No Matter the Distance* by Cindy Baldwin (New York: HarperCollins, 2023)
- *The Year Life Went Down the Toilet* by Jake Maia Arlow (New York: Dial Books, 2023)
- *Wednesday & Woof: Catastrophe* by Sherri Winston (New York: HarperCollins, 2022)
- *Wink* by Rob Harrell (New York: Dial Books, 2020)

Communication

- *Brayden Speaks Up* by Brayden Harrington and Betty C. Tang (New York: Harper, 2021)

- *I Talk Like a River* by Jordan Scott and Sydney Smith (London: Walker Books Ltd., 2020)
- *Phone Call with a Fish* by Silvia Vecchini and Sualzo (Grand Rapids: Eerdmans Books for Young Readers, 2018)
- Speechless by Aron Nels Steinke (New York: Scholastic, Graphix, 2025)
- *Talking Is Not My Thing* by Rose Robbins (Grand Rapids: Eerdmans Books for Young Readers, 2020)
- This Is How We Talk: A Celebration of Disability and Connection by Jessica Slice, Caroline Cupp, and Kayla Harren (New York: Dial Books, 2025)

Hearing Disabilities

- *Can Bears Ski?* by Raymond Antrobus and Polly Dunbar (Somerville, MA: Candlewick Press, 2020)
- *Dancing Hands: A Story of Friendship in Filipino Sign Language* by Joanna Que, Charina Marquez, and Fran Alvarez (San Francisco: Chronicle Books, 2023)
- *El Deafo* by Cece Bell (New York: Amulet Books, 2014)
- *Listen: How Evelyn Glennie, a Deaf Girl, Changed Percussion* by Shannon Stocker and Devon Holzwarth (New York: Dial Books, 2022)
- *Next Door* by Deborah Kerbel and Isaac Liang (Toronto: Kids Can Press, 2023)
- *Show Me a Sign* by Ann Clare LeZotte (New York: Scholastic Press, 2020)
- *The Fastest Girl on Earth: Meet Kitty O'Neil, Daredevil Driver!* by Dean Robbins and Elizabeth Baddeley (New York: Knopf, 2021)
- *The William Hoy Story: How a Deaf Baseball Player Changed the Game* by Nancy Churin and Jez Tuya (Park Ridge, IL: Albert Whitman & Company, 2016)

Intellectual and Developmental Disabilities

- *I Am a Masterpiece: An Empowering Story About Inclusivity and Growing Up with Down Syndrome* by Mia Armstrong, Marissa Moss, and Alexandra Thompson (New York: Random House Children's Books, 2024)
- *The Unstoppable Jamie* by Joy Givens and Courtney Dawson (New York: Two Lions, 2023)
- *Unbound: The Life + Art of Judith Scott* by Joyce Scott, Brie Spangler, and Melissa Sweet (New York: Knopf, 2021)

Learning Disabilities

- *Aaron Slater, Illustrator* by Andrea Beaty and David Roberts (New York: Abrams Books for Young Readers, 2021)
- *Abdul's Story* by Jamilah Thompkins-Bigelow and Tiffany Rose (New York: Simon & Schuster Books for Young Readers, 2022)
- *Ben & Emma's Big Hit* by Gavin Newsom, Ruby Shamir, and Alexandra Thompson (New York: Philomel, 2021)
- *Figure It Out, Henri Weldon* by Tanita S. Davis (New York: Katherine Tegen Books, 2023)
- *Fish in a Tree* by Lynda Mullaly Hunt (London: Puffin Books, 2017)
- *I Do Not Like Books Anymore!* by Daisy Hirst (Somerville, MA: Candlewick Press, 2018)
- *Thank You, Mr. Falker* by Patricia Polacco (New York: Philomel Books, 1998)
- *The Extra-Special Group* —Hey Jack! Series by Sally Rippin (San Diego: Kane Miller, 2020)
- *The Junkyard Wonders* by Patricia Polacco (New York: Philomel Books, 2010)
- *Welcome Back, Maple Mehta-Cohen: A Story for Anyone Who Has Ever Felt Different* by Kate McGovern (Somerville, MA: Candlewick Press, 2023)
- *Wiggling Words: Loving Language with Dyslexia* by Kate Rolfe (Somerville, MA: Candlewick Press, 2026)

Mental Health

- *A Blue Kind of Day* by Rachel Tomlinson and Tori-Jay Mordey (New York: Kokila, 2022)
- *A Voice in the Storm* by Karl James Mountford (Somerville, MA: Candlewick Studio, 2024)
- *Alvin Ho: Allergic to Camping, Hiking, and Other Natural Disasters* by Lenore Look and Leuyen Pham (New York: Yearling, 2009)
- *Cranky* by Phuc Tran and Pete Oswald (New York: Harper, 2024)
- *Dark Cloud* by Anna Lazowski and Penny Neville-Lee (Toronto: Kids Can Press, 2023)
- *How to Tantrum Like a Champion: Ten Small Ways to Temper Big Feelings* by Allan Wolf and Keisha Morris (Somerville, MA: Candlewick Press, 2024)

- *I Think I Think a Lot* by Jessica Whipple and Josée Bisaillon (Minneapolis: Free Spirit Publishing, 2024)
- *It's So Difficult* by Guridi (Grand Rapids, MI: Eerdman Books for Young Readers, 2022)
- *Invisible Isabel* by Sally J. Pla and Tania de Regil (New York: Quill Tree Books, 2024)
- *Loud!* by Rose Robbins (London: Scallywag Press Ltd., 2023)
- *Millie and Me* by Lauren Castillo (Somerville, MA: Candlewick Press, 2024)
- *My Thoughts Have Wings* by Maggie Smith and Leanne Hatch (New York: Balzer + Bray, 2024)
- *Octopus Moon* by Bobbie Pyron (New York: Nancy Paulsen Books, 2025)
- *Puzzled* by Pan Cooke (New York: Rocky Pond Books, 2024)
- *Sensitive* by Sara Levine and Mehrdokht Amini (Minneapolis, Carolrhoda, 2023)
- *The Cat Who Couldn't Be Bothered* by Jack Kurland (Beverly, MA: Frances Lincoln Children's Books, 2024)
- *The Poet and the Bees* by Amy Novesky and Jessica Love (New York: Viking Books for Young Readers, 2025)
- *The Worry (Less) Book: Feel Strong, Find Calm, and Tame Your Anxiety* by Rachel Brian (New York: Little, Brown and Company, 2020)
- *Today* by Gavi Snyder and Stephanie Graegin (New York: A Paula Wiseman Book, 2024)
- *What to Do When You Worry Too Much: A Kid's Guide to Overcoming Anxiety* by Dawn Huebner, PhD and Bonnie Matthews (Washington, DC: Magination Press, 2021)
- *When Sadness Is at Your Door* by Eva Eland (New York: Random House, 2019)

Neurodivergence

- *A Boy Called Bat* by Elana K. Arnold and Charles Santos (New York: Walden Pond Press, 2017)
- *A Day with No Words* by Tiffany Hammond and Kate Cosgrove (New Egypt, NJ: Wheat Penny Press, 2023)

- *A Tale as Tall as Jacob: Misadventures with My Brother* by Samantha Edwards (Kansas City, MO: Andrews McMeel Publishing, 2021)
- *All the Small Wonderful Things* by Kate Foster (Somerville, MA: Candlewick Press, 2025)
- *Can You See Me* by Libby Scott and Rebecca Westcott (New York: Scholastic, 2020)
- *Charlie Makes a Splash!* by Holly Robinson Peete, RJ Peete, and Shane W. Evans (New York: Scholastic Press, 2022)
- *Each Tiny Spark* by Pablo Cartaya (New York: Kokila, 2019)
- *Flap Your Hands: A Celebration of Stimming* by Steve Asbell (New York: Lee & Low Books, 2024)
- *Frankie's World* by Aoife Dooley (New York: Graphix, 2022)
- *Gina Kaminski Saves the Wolf* by Craig Barr-Green and Francis Martin (San Diego: Kane Miler, 2024)
- *Good Different* by Meg Eden Kuyatt (New York: Scholastic Press, 2023)
- *Harriet Hound* by Kate Foster and Sophie Beer (Somerville, MA: Candlewick Press, 2024)
- *Henry and the Something New* by Jenn Bailey and Mika Song (San Francisco: Chronicle Books, 2024)
- *Henry's Picture-Perfect Day* by Jenn Bailey and Mika Song (San Francisco: Chronicle Books, 2025)
- *How Are You, Verity?* by Meghan Wilson Duff and Taylor Barron (Washington, DC: Magination Press, 2023)
- *It Was Supposed to Be Sunny* by Samantha Cotterill (New York: Dial Books for Young Readers, 2021)
- *Jay and Ben* by Lulu Delacre and Katharine Swanson (New York: Lee & Low Books, 2011)
- *Leo and the Octopus* by Isabelle Marinov and Chris Nixon (San Diego: Kane Miller, 2021)
- *My Brain Is Magic: A Sensory-Seeking Celebration* (Minneapolis: Soaring Kite Books, 2023)
- *Next Level: A Hymn in Gratitude for Neurodiversity* by Samara Cole Doyon and Kaylani Juanita (Ann Arbor, MI: Tilbury House, 2024)

- *Nope. Never. Not for Me!* by Samantha Cotterill (New York: Dial Books for Young Readers, 2019)
- *Rissy No Kissies* by Katey Howes and Jess Engle (Minneapolis: Carolrhoda Books, 2021)
- *Speak Up!* by Rebecca Burgess (New York: Quill Tree Books, 2022)
- *That Always Happens Sometimes* by Kiley Frnak and K-Fai Steele (New York: Knopf Books for Young Readers, 2024)
- *The Boy with the Butterfly Mind* by Victoria Williamson (Edinburgh, UK: Kelpies, 2019)
- *The Spectrum Girl's Survival Guide: How to Grow Up Awesome and Autistic* by Siena Castellon (London: Jessica Kingsley Publishers, 2020)
- *The View from the Very Best House in Town* by Meera Trehan (Somerville, MA: Candlewick Press, 2022)
- *Too Much! An Overwhelming Day* by Jolene Gutiérrez and Angel Chang (New York: Abrams Appleseed, 2023)
- *Too Sticky! Sensory Issues with Autism* by Jen Malia and Joanne Lew-Vriethoff (Chicago: Albert Whitman & Company, 2020)
- *We Could Be Heroes* by Margaret Finnegan (New York: Atheneum Books, 2020)
- *Wepa* by J de laVega (Los Angeles: Little Libros, 2023)
- *Wonderfully Wired Brains: An Introduction to the World of Neurodiversity* by Louise Gooding and Ruth Burrows (New York: DK Publishing, 2023)

Physical Disabilities

- *All the Way to the Top: How One Girl's Fight with Disabilities Changed Everything* by Annette Bay Pimentel and Nabi H. Ali (Naperville, IL: Sourcebooks eXplore, 2020)
- *Dorothea's Eyes* by Barb Rosenstock and Gérard DuBois (Honesdale, PA: Calkins Creek, 2016)
- *I Will Dance* by Nancy Bo Flood and Julianna Swaney (New York: Atheneum Books for Young Readers, 2020)
- *Knockin' On Wood: Starring Peg Leg Bates* by Lynne Barasch (New York: Lee & Low Books, 2004)

- *Lucas at the Paralympics* by Igor Plohl, Urška Stropnik Šonc, and Nika Lopert (New York: Holiday House, 2018)

- *Rescue and Jessica: A Life-Changing Friendship* (Somerville, MA: Candlewick Press, 2018)

- *Roll with It* by Jamie Sumner (New York: Atheneum Books for Young Readers, 2019)

- *Sam's Super Seats* by Keah Brown and Sharee Miller (New York: Kokila, 2022)

- *Splash* by Claire Cashmore and Sharon Davey (San Diego: Kane Miller, 2022)

- *Stay Curious: A Brief History of Stephen Hawking* by Kathleen Krull, Paul Brewer, and Boris Kulikov (New York: Crown Books for Young Readers, 2020)

- *Tenacious: Fifteen Adventures Alongside Disabled Athletes* by Patty Cisneros Prevo and Dion MBD (New York: Lee & Low Books, 2023)

- *The War That Saved My Life* by Kimberly Brubaker Bradley (London: Puffin Books, 2015)

- *We Move Together* by Kelly Fritsch, Anne McGuire, and Eduardo Trejos (Chico, CA: AK Press, 2021)

- *What Happened to You?* by James Catchpole and Karen George (New York: Little, Brown and Company, 2021)

- *Zimmy: The Human Fish* by David A. Adler and Rob Shepperson (New York: Holiday House, 2026)

Vision

- *A Sky That Sings* by Anita Sanchez, George Steele, and Emily Mendoza (New York: Lee & Low Books, 2025)

- *Cakes and Miracles: A Purim Tale* by Barbara Diamond Goldin and Jaime Zollars (Tarrytown, NY: Marshall Cavendish Children, 2010)

- *My City Speaks* by Darren Lebeuf and Ashley Barron (Toronto: Kids Can Press, 2021)

- *Ray Charles* by Sharon Bell Mathis and George Ford (New York: Lee & Low Books, 2001)

> **TIP** The National Library Services (NLS) for the Blind and Print Disabled offers access to thousands of materials in audio and electronic braille. NLS provides reading materials at *no cost* to people who are blind, deaf-blind, visually impaired, have a physical disability, or a reading disability that makes reading regular print challenging. Once registered, your child can access texts with a talking-book player or through the BARD Mobile app on their personal electronic device.

BEYOND THIS LIST

This list isn't exhaustive. Despite spending months combing the shelves of my local library and working with several children's publishers, I know I may have missed some recently published books that feature disabled characters. And, of course, many more books will be in print by the time this book is in your hands.

Over the past decade, picture book illustrators have intentionally shown more racial, religious, and ethnic diversity in their books. Often, background characters have a range of skin colors or might wear a yarmulke or hijab. In addition, illustrators will represent disabilities by showing someone using a white cane, sitting in a wheelchair, or wearing a hearing aid. Those books matter since they are mirrors for some children! However, I intentionally shared books that centered on disabilities rather than just showing a character with a visible disability. Many disabilities and chronic medical conditions are invisible, so I looked beyond illustrations-only and examined the actual text of the books too.

The internet abounds with book lists. Here are three you might check out to extend my list.

The **American Library Association (ALA)** has many book awards, including the Schneider Family Book Award. This award "honors an author or illustrator for a book that embodies an artistic expression of the disability experience for child and adolescent audiences." (See Resources.)

The **International Board on Books for Young People (IBBY)** curates a collection of books for young people with disabilities annually. You can use their list to continue curating more books for your child. (See Resources.)

Social Justice Books has nearly 100 book lists that are constantly being updated. They provide lists that aren't only current but also curated with care toward marginalized groups. (See Resources.)

Many book influencers curate lists and share them online. Those on Instagram are often called Bookstagrammers, while those on TikTok may be called BookTok creators. Bookstagrammers and BookTok creators can be resources for new titles released after *this* book's publication.

PRACTICAL TIPS FOR READING WITH YOUR CHILD

As you read, you'll encounter places where you want to think or talk. You can prompt your child to think more deeply about the characters, setting, or presented information. More often than not, you'll want to ask questions to ensure your child understands the book. There are ways to teach reading skills—like envisioning, inferring, and prediction—just by turning and talking to your child.

Engagement Strategies to Use While Reading

Children learn more when they talk, so it's imperative to take the time to practice conversations about the text with your child. This will help them process it alongside you. We can attend to our children by engaging in conversations about books. One way to do this is by removing disruptions, like cell phones, from the space. Another way we can focus is by leaning in, making eye contact (if that's comfortable for your child), and asking questions.

Here are some sentence stems to help support your child's oral language *while* reading and talking about a book with you. Some of these might be helpful to you and your child, while others may be too advanced. Use the ones that feel developmentally appropriate for your child.

- Another example is . . .
- Another reason is . . .
- Could it also be that . . .
- For example . . .
- Have you considered . . .
- I noticed that section, too . . . and I think this connects to the whole story because . . .
- I partly agree but . . . because . . .
- I see (the item you are discussing), and then a similar thing happens (in this place), I think this is repeated because . . .
- I think this is important because . . .
- I used to think . . . but now I'm realizing . . .

- In the beginning . . . then later . . . finally . . .
- In the beginning . . . in the middle . . . at the end . . .
- Many people think . . . but I think . . .
- Might the reason for this be . . .
- On the other hand . . .
- The reason for this is . . .
- There is one thing in the story that doesn't "fit" for me and it's . . .
- This connects with . . .
- This differs from . . .
- This is different from . . .
- This is giving me the idea that . . .
- This is important because . . .
- This makes me realize . . .
- This might be present because . . .
- This is similar to . . .
- What makes you think [this]?

Engagement Strategies to Use after Reading

Most adults want to talk to someone after reading a book. This is why book clubs exist! Some books include discussion group questions at the back of the book to help members spark meaningful discussions. Sometimes reading and discussing a text leads to the next book club choice, which can be an outgrowth of reading the author's note at the back of the book. As a result, you can continue to use the sentence starters in the previous section to have a book talk with your child *after* you're finished reading.

If you want to take things further, you can discuss the text with a critical literacy lens. *Critical literacy* is a thinking skill that involves questioning, analyzing, interpreting, and responding to texts since they are socially constructed from distinct perspectives. On the most basic level, critical literacy allows us to consider multiple perspectives, examine whose voice is privileged, and who might be marginalized or silenced.

When I taught fifth grade in the New York City Public Schools, I compiled critical listening questions for my fifth graders and me to use with read-aloud books. Here are several questions I used with my students that you can weave into book chats with your child as you read.

- How is the author using power in this text? Does the author use his or her power to repeat stereotypes or challenge them?
- What are the ways this text can be challenged?
- What is privileged in this text?
- What is the purpose of the text?
- What power relations might the author have had to negotiate through the publishing of this text?
- What view of the world is put forth by the ideas in this text? What views are not?
- What are the other possible constructions of the world?
- Who is seen in this text? Who isn't represented in this text?
- Who, or what, benefits from the power in the text?
- Who, or what, would not benefit from the power in this text?
- Whose interests are served by the dissemination of this text? Whose interests are not served?

You might be tempted to take your conversation further because your child is excited about a book. In that case, you could co-write a book review. Book reviews can be written or spoken. They can be as simple as writing a review on Goodreads or StoryGraph or as complex as a recorded booktalk shared with people (such as classmates or family members) whom you and your child think would appreciate it.

Sometimes a book is just a book. You can preplan by using some of the sentence stems in this chapter, or you can just wing it. Either option is okay! After all, reading alongside your child is a fantastic way to bond.

ENCOURAGE YOUR CHILD TO SEEK OUT DIVERSE BOOKS

I hope your child will love trips to the library or the bookstore as they grow. Introduce your child to the children's librarian or your local bookseller. These people know books so well. If needed, facilitate the conversations to help your child communicate the kinds of books they enjoy or want to read. I've found librarians and booksellers truly care about kids reading and want to match them with the best possible books to help them become lifelong readers.

My daughter began to enjoy reading when she was 10 years old. She identified several authors whose books she liked and began looking for their new releases by perusing Apple Books for soon-to-be-released books. Even though she'd be far beyond the reading level of a beloved book series, she'd return to it between the middle-grade novels she was reading. She'd quickly zoom through those books and return to something on her present reading level once she finished each one. At 14, she no longer returns to those beloved series, but she still takes the initiative to self-select books, which matters.

Halfway through middle school, something else started happening. Suddenly, she was seeking out diverse books that were mirrors for her. She read books with characters who had similar non-apparent disabilities or health conditions. She located books with characters who shared our religion. She even found a book with a character who was trying to tame her curly hair, just like she was. Being able to step back and watch her seek out books where she saw herself was a big moment. I occasionally offer gentle suggestions for finding window and sliding doors books, but I notice she makes excellent choices about books independently.

Having the opportunity and choice to self-select books empowers kids as readers. As we move into the next chapter, we look at another way to strengthen your child by teaching them how to self-advocate.

Tip for Cultivating Joy: Get to know the resources at your local library. The library's collection extends beyond the books you see in the stacks. You can access audiobooks, ebooks, magazines, and more through apps like Libby and Hoopla with a library card. Discovering new authors, genres, or series—whether for yourself or your child—can spark curiosity and bring moments of joy into your everyday life.

Self-Care Tip: Try to carve out time for a reading life rather than reading only on vacation or putting it off until your child is older. Find time to read what you love daily . . . even if it's only 10 minutes before bedtime. Remember, all reading counts, so read what brings you happiness!

10

Teach Self-Advocacy

Teaching young children to advocate for themselves is challenging! However, it is crucial to provide opportunities for your child to speak up for themselves, express their needs, and make decisions that impact their lives. Self-advocacy is a process that involves:

- Knowing yourself and your context
- Knowing your rights and responsibilities
- Building communication skills and strategies
- Collaborating and leading with others

Every child should become a confident self-advocate. For children with disabilities, these skills enable them to seek assistance, express their needs, manage unfair situations, and develop negotiation and problem-solving abilities. Studies indicate that elementary school-aged children with disabilities need to understand themselves and their rights to communicate and advocate for themselves and for others effectively. I've modified a conceptual framework designed by Test and Colleagues to demonstrate what K-6 students can achieve as self-advocates, shown on page 170.

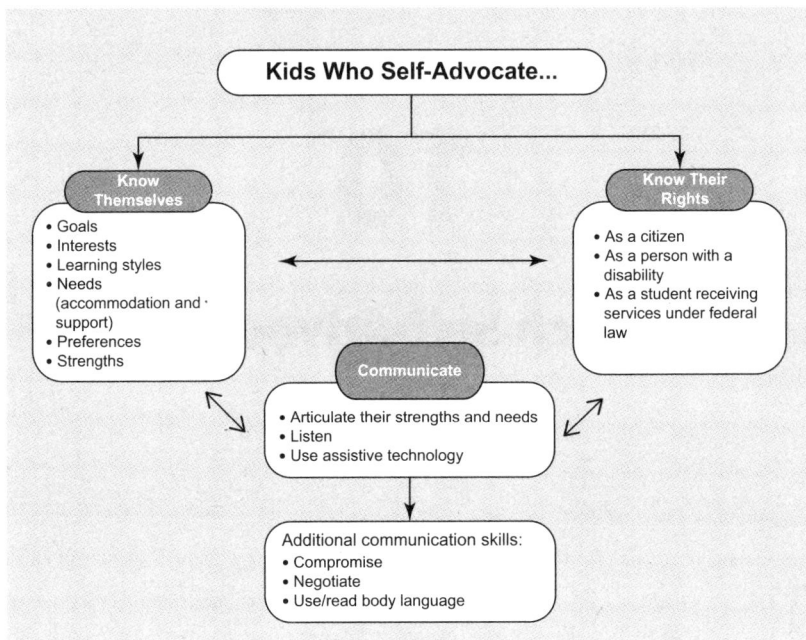

From Test et al. (2005). Adapted by permission.

When my daughter was in elementary school, I often advocated for her needs. Even though she had the communication skills to speak up, she often felt too shy or scared to advocate for herself. Unfortunately, I didn't start to work with her on self-advocacy skills until sixth grade. Now, as a teenager, she is such an effective self-advocate that I coach her, but I rarely need to step in. What I should have known then that I know now is that we must be in the business of putting ourselves out of a job. Not only does passing this torch relieve us of problem solving for our kids all the time, but it also gives our children the gift of self-determination, the power of authority over their current circumstances and future aspirations.

COMMON CHALLENGES

Children with disabilities may face challenges in three main areas—academic, physical, and social-emotional contexts. These challenges often intersect and compound each other, creating complex barriers for K–6 children with disabilities. It's helpful to identify where your child may need the most help so they can focus their self-advocacy efforts where they'll produce the most significant benefit. Some challenges they may encounter include, but are not limited to:

Academic Challenges

- Attention and focus can manifest as difficulty concentrating or staying on task.
- Communication challenges may manifest as expressing thoughts clearly, understanding directions, and more.
- Learning difficulties may manifest in reading, writing, math, or other academic subjects.
- Memory issues might cause trouble retaining or recalling information.
- Slower processing speed means it takes a child longer to comprehend and respond to information.

Physical Challenges

- Fatigue and reduced stamina mean a child tires more quickly than peers during physical activities.
- Fine motor skill deficits might include difficulty with writing, buttoning clothing, or using utensils.
- Health issues might be ongoing and require frequent medical appointments or treatments.
- Mobility limitations make it difficult for a child to move independently or access certain areas of the school.
- Sensory processing issues might manifest as oversensitivity or undersensitivity to sensory stimuli.

Social and Emotional Challenges

- Anger and frustration might stem from difficulties in various areas of life—in or out of school.
- Anxiety and depression are two mental health issues that can impact many aspects of a child's life.
- Bullying or social isolation might mean that a student is a target of teasing or exclusion by peers.
- Emotional regulation issues could mean a student struggles to manage their feelings or respond appropriately to situations.
- Low self-esteem can manifest as inadequacy or a negative perception of oneself.
- Social skill deficits make it harder for a child to interpret social cues or engage in age-appropriate interactions.

SELF-ADVOCACY SKILLS AND STRATEGIES

Numerous challenges can be tackled or lessened through accommodations, appropriate support, and interventions, allowing children to thrive and develop their abilities to navigate tricky situations. Moreover, when children successfully navigate challenges independently—despite their difficulty—they gain greater confidence in their capacity to tackle tough things.

The following strategies can support their self-advocacy where they need it.

Getting Used to Asking for What They Need

All kids have needs, and they'll have to ask for some assistance. Teaching them self-advocacy should start with helping them get comfortable speaking up in general. Some children know what they need or want but are too shy to speak up, while others are still learning what they need to be successful in school. Learning self-advocacy doesn't happen overnight.

One of the most important things we can do for children is help them become comfortable talking to adults. This starts with small conversations with neighbors, in your house of worship, or in a medical waiting room. It can also involve having your child order their meal or request something (like more water or a dessert menu) at a restaurant. As kids grow more comfortable communicating with other adults alongside you, there's a greater chance they'll be comfortable enough with their teacher to advocate for themselves.

Another way to help your child develop confidence in advocating for themselves is to rehearse scenarios they might encounter at school. I've always been a big *let's practice this at home* person. Rehearsing goes a long way since it allows a child to work out the kinks in their message and adjust their pacing. As a parent, you can move your child closer to independence if you rehearse scenarios at home, like requesting:

- A second explanation when something is unclear
- More time to complete an assignment
- Use of the restroom
- Use of the calm-down corner or a break
- To work with a different partner/group

See the box below for three ways to boost self-advocacy skills at home.

Three Things You Can Do at Home to Increase Your Child's Self-Confidence

- **Model problem solving**: Demonstrate how to address issues calmly and effectively with other household members. Unpack how you solved a problem after you modeled it, and allow your child to ask questions to clarify how you worked things out.
- **Practice scenarios**: Role-play potential challenging situations to help your child prepare responses. Providing home practice time allows kids to find the right words in a difficult situation.
- **Offer choices**: Give your child opportunities to make decisions to provide practice in responsible decision making and foster a sense of autonomy.

Your child must learn to get the teacher's attention and ask for what they need. Cards can be printed for children who need the teacher's attention but are afraid to speak up. Examples include "I need a break right now" and "I need help with . . . " Having a child request something with a preprinted card demonstrates that they can problem-solve in the moment to help them get what they need.

Amy Fisher of The Arc Lancaster Lebanon has created "advocacy cheat sheets" for some elementary school students she has worked with. To make them, Amy:

- Asks kids what is important for people to know about them
- Then asks the child how they communicate what they need
- Simultaneously speaks with the child's parent to get their input
- Records how the child feels others can help them

Kids can then refer to these customized sheets for the proper verbiage to communicate their needs. A short and a longer version are shown on pages 174–175.

One-Page Profile

My Name _____

What's important for people to know?

How I communicate what I need.

How to best support ME.

What Do I Need?

My Name _____

Personal

☐ I need a quiet space when things get too noisy and busy.

☐ I need you to give me time to process what you say to me.

☐ I need to be included in the fun.

☐ I need you to talk directly to me and not to my aide or my parents.

☐ I need you to understand my support needs.

School

☐ I need activities that are meaningful and engaging.

☐ I need the people who support me to understand how I learn and communicate.

☐ I need direct instruction, lots of repetition, the opportunity for breaks, and tasks broken down into smaller, manageable steps.

☐ I need to be with my peers.

Health

☐ I need my teachers and paras to understand how I communicate pain and discomfort.

☐ I need to have someone take care of my toileting needs in a way that is comfortable and respects my privacy.

☐ I need to visit the nurse for medication per my doctor's schedule.

Other

☐ Ask me before you move my chair.

☐ Communicate what you are doing when you must change my position or physically touch me.

☐ Remember that I communicate differently but still have things I want, need, like, and dislike.

☐ Don't be afraid to ask someone for help if you don't understand what I'm trying to communicate.

You can also involve your child in the creation of an informational sheet (You might call it "A Little About Me"), as I did with my daughter and as shown below, to share at an initial or annual IEP meeting. You can include a recent photo. A sheet like this personalizes your child, so they take part in showing the IEP team who they are. Another type of information sheet, which can also be used for the purpose of IEP planning, is shown in Chapter 7.

A Little about Me

Personal Information

Name

Birthday

Who I live with

Favorite Things

Book genre

Game

Sport

Subject

What I Did this Summer

My Strengths

My biggest academic strengths are:

Ways You Can Help Me

Things I'm Working On

Some of my biggest challenges are:

Self-Advocacy Language

Some students are nervous about approaching grown-ups because they're shy, anxious, have limited expressive language, or might be learning English as a second language. Whatever the case, they need phrases to help them get started. Lean sentence starters can be given to students to help them practice speaking up. See the box below, also available to download and print at *www.guilford.com/shubitz-materials* for use with your child.

Sentence Starters Your Child Can Use to Build Self-Advocacy at School

1. Can I speak to you privately/in the hallway?
2. I'm feeling confused about . . .
3. I'm worried about . . . Can we discuss it?
4. I need help with . . . Could you help me?
5. I'm having trouble with . . . Can you assist me?
6. I'm struggling with . . . Can we talk about it?
7. I'm not sure how to . . . Could you show me again?
8. Can you please check if I understood the instructions correctly?
9. Can you please slow down? I'm having trouble keeping up.
10. I'm not comfortable with . . . Is there another way I can do this?

You, too, can use certain language to help your child build self-advocacy skills. Most kids don't elaborate when asked, "How was your day?" but there are other questions you can ask (see the box on pages 177–178) to find out how the school day went.

Questions That Will Help Your Child Understand Where Help Might Be Needed

- What was the most challenging thing you had to do today?
- What strengths did you use during the school day?

- Did you learn anything challenging or confusing?
- What positive choices did you make at school?
- Did you feel frustrated with anything today?
- How did you show your best self at school today?

Coaching Academic Self-Advocacy

Your child's Individualized Education Program (IEP) provides valuable insight into their academic challenges. Teachers and service providers should communicate these IEP goals to your child in *kid-friendly language,* ensuring they understand what they're working toward. This doesn't always happen, so it's important that *you* review your child's IEP goals with them. You can build in a regular time, such as when you receive their progress-monitoring reports, to review your child's goals with them so they know what they're trying to get better at as a learner.

> Be sure to go over IEP goals with your child to ensure that your child knows when something new has been added.

Your child should be taught about their IEP. Knowing their accommodations, modifications, and services will empower kids to advocate for themselves if they're not happening or being provided regularly.

Accommodations are designed to make the general curriculum accessible to your child, although IEP goals don't always directly drive day-to-day classroom instruction. These goals sometimes measure progress in areas separate from the general education classroom's activities. While accommodations support learning, they aren't directly tied to the IEP goals that measure the continued need for special education services.

Identifying Academic Challenges

It's hard, but empowering, to admit when schoolwork becomes challenging. Kids need to know that *it's okay to ask for help*. We can work with our children at home to give them this language because their school may or may not be teaching this well. Some key phrases include the following:

- I don't understand this . . .
- I don't know where to start. Can you help me with that?
- I tried this, and I'm still confused. Please help me.

Examples of how to ask for specific help when your child needs certain accommodations are in the table below.

Asking for Specific Help

For an accommodation like this . . .	Your child can ask for help like this . . .
Pair text-to-speech, or TTS, or audiobooks with printed material	"Do you have this as an audiobook?" "Can I open my tablet and use TTS for this?"
Chunk larger assignments into smaller tasks	"How long should I work on this today?" "What am I responsible for completing this period?" "Can I have a checklist to use?"
Use a frequency modulation, or FM, system to amplify the teacher's voice and reduce background noise	"Can you put on the mic so I can hear you better?" "Would you bring the FM system to {PE, music, art,} so I can hear the other teachers?"
Give the option to type assignments that are more than one paragraph	"May I use my tablet for this assignment?" "Can I go to {quiet place} to use speech-to-text, or STT, as I type?"

If your child isn't comfortable speaking up at school but reports problems with receiving designated accommodations to you—such as not getting tests read to them or not having seen the guidance counselor in three weeks—reach out to your child's case manager. Consider having your child sit beside you when you compose a message asking for more information. Witnessing your advocacy for their needs will help them learn how to self-advocate in the future.

Championing Physical Needs

Children with physical disabilities need to speak up to help the adults in school understand, "This is what I need." Kids need to know that they have rights as a protected class and that what might seem basic to someone else can be crucial to them. Some examples include the following:

- **Assistive Technology:** An AAC device, adapted keyboard, adjustable touch screen stylus, screen reader, and tablet mounting system are some of the many pieces of technology kids can use to participate fully in the educational environment.

- **Mobility:** An adult might help a child with mobility challenges navigate the hallways safely, help them with toileting, or assist them at recess so they can engage with their peers on adapted playground equipment.

- **Sensory:** Students can access fidgets, lower lighting, noise-canceling headphones, quiet rooms, and sensory breaks whenever needed.

The Restroom

As a teacher, I kept my minilesson times short but sacred, and all students were expected to be in the classroom. If students missed the instruction, they would be confused when they returned, and someone—another student or I—would have to catch them up. It was a huge waste of time! As a result, my students planned their restroom trips before or after the lesson.

Here's the thing: Sometimes, you've got to go! As a classroom teacher, I never wanted students to get to the point where they danced before me to keep their bodily fluids in. As a result, I'd allow more than one kid into the bathroom at a time (In many schools, an unwritten rule is that no more than one boy or one girl is out at a time.) if they needed to go. I always told them I'd have their back.

If you have a kid who has to use the restroom more than the average person or has accidents because they wait too long, you must inform the teacher as soon as possible. If the teacher knows that your child needs to use the restroom frequently, they can ask to use the bathroom and know that their request will be granted. If needed, you can ask your family doctor to write a medical note about bathroom frequency and have an SDI put into the IEP that allows your child to use the restroom when requested.

Social and Emotional Advocacy

Social and emotional learning, or SEL, comes up in conversation and news more frequently every year—and for good reason. Children's social and emotional needs must be met; otherwise, learning and retaining information will be difficult or impossible. SEL is designed to help kids learn and practice skills that will prepare them for academic success and help them develop and maintain healthy relationships, be productive members of society, and have fulfilling careers.

The Collaborative for Academic, Social, and Emotional Learning, or CASEL, developed a framework that includes five core competencies for SEL. Their video *SEL 101: What are the core competencies and key settings?* defines the competency areas as follows:

1. **Self-awareness** helps children develop a sense of who they are.
2. **Self-management** teaches children how to manage stress.
3. **Social awareness** instructs children to understand the views of others.
4. **Relationship skills** provide skills for connecting and engaging with other people.
5. **Responsible decision making** shows students how to make caring and considerate choices.

CASEL asserts that SEL works best when evidence-based programs are implemented and students are trusted partners in their learning. (See the Resources for evidence-based programs.) I believe that progress can be made when parents and schools work together to forge students' social and emotional development. Strong family partnerships, like the ones you're building with your child's teachers and service providers, will aid their social and emotional growth.

Sometimes the SEL acronym is used too flippantly, lumping together social and emotional skills that are distinct in important ways:

- **Social Skills:** Help children interact positively with others. They learn to establish and grow relationships and make responsible decisions.

- **Emotional Skills:** Guide children to recognize their emotions, handle their feelings, and effectively manage their emotional responses.

What You Can Expect from Your Child's School

Instruction in these fundamental skills is essential. But how do you get it for your child? And how can your child self-advocate for their social and emotional needs? As with academic and physical challenges, you may have to be your child's first advocate at the start (and even going forward), but your child can learn important self-advocacy skills *through* SEL provided in school. SEL offerings vary from school to school, so you may have to ask the school, "How are you teaching my child the SEL skills they need?" or "How do you know the emotional capacity of the students?" If the school can't point to a methodology or share its curriculum, you could advocate for the adoption of one. You'll find resources for exploring SEL at the back of the book.

> Just as each state develops academic standards (that are often similar to those contained in the Common Core State Standards Initiative), states can write their own social and emotional learning standards. Many states use the CASEL framework and resources when formulating their SEL standards.

Social Skills Instruction

Many schools devote time to social skills essential for strong interpersonal relationships. Ideally, social skills instruction should occur in the general education setting since all students need to work on communication, conflict resolution, emotional regulation, and problem solving. Deliberate social skills instruction is often given during a morning meeting, an advisory period, after recess, in a closing circle, or during other dedicated SEL time, which might be called a *brain break* or a *body break*.

In some schools, social skills are explicitly taught to children in small groups outside the classroom to help them build and sustain relationships. Some of this direct instruction includes role-playing everyday social situations, like joining a game at recess or asking for help. Students also practice circles of communication to help them make small talk in the lunchroom. Through social skills support, students learn that kindness, sharing, and listening are keys to building friendships.

If your child struggles with interpersonal communication, you can advocate for more explicit social skills instruction within the school day. (The school will determine if your child qualifies for this. If they do, this can be written into your child's IEP.)

Recognizing Emotional Needs

It's vital to help children identify their emotions since unaddressed emotional issues can manifest as academic, behavioral, or social challenges. You can foster self-advocacy skills at home by creating opportunities for your child to practice communication and problem solving. This approach can be particularly beneficial for children who exhibit different behaviors at home than at school. To encourage advocacy at home, you can:

- **Initiate conversations:** Regularly engage your child in discussions about their day, feelings, and needs. Consider drawing or playing while talking with your child so these conversations don't feel like interrogations.

- **Create a soft place to land:** Establish an environment where your child feels comfortable expressing themselves without fear of judgment or concern that you'll be angry at them. You might use some of the following phrases:

  ○ I hear you and understand you're frustrated/scared/upset right now.

  ○ I notice your heart is racing. Let's go to our calm-down space together.

  ○ I see you're frustrated/scared/upset. Can you tell me what happened?

  ○ You are always safe with me.

  ○ Your feelings matter. It's good to share them with others.

  ○ I love you.

- **Teach emotional vocabulary:** Help your child identify and articulate their emotions accurately. This helps kids understand nuances rather than relying on umbrella terms like *happy, sad,* and *mad.* (See Resources.)

- **Encourage alternatives to meltdowns:** Guide your child to verbalize their needs instead of resorting to emotional outbursts. Kids should know when they need a break and why it's helpful to them. Help your child understand what triggers their need for a break and then encourage them to ask, "Can I have a break now?" This can feel daunting to an elementary school-aged child to do at school, so helping your child to ask for a break before they get overstimulated at home and when you're out in the community can be a gateway to teaching them how to ask before they feel triggered or begin to unravel at school.

- **Validate feelings:** Acknowledge your child's emotions while helping them find constructive ways to express them. Art, music, physical activity, outdoor play, and being in nature can help children express their feelings constructively.

- **Establish routines:** To help your child feel more in control, create a predictable home environment. Checklists and visual schedules can make routines, such as getting ready for bed or what to take to school daily, more concrete. A visual schedule can make challenging times, like getting ready for school, packing a lunch, or recalling items to take home at the end of the day, less stressful. For younger children, pair words with images. You can use clipart or take photos of your child's actual belongings (for example, their toothbrush, pajamas, book basket, and bed if you're creating a bedtime chart). Making these charts will assist your kids with routines—and it will likely encourage them to become list-makers as they grow older.

- **Managing emotions:** Provide your child with various calm-down options (such as a calm-down jar, a weighted blanket, a body sock, blowing bubbles, repeating a mantra) to help them learn how to manage strong emotions independently. In addition, you can help your child learn to identify their feelings and tell someone when they're feeling angry. When they're ready, children can use *I* statements to communicate their feelings.

- **Celebrate successes:** Recognize and praise instances when the child effectively advocates for themselves and their needs.

Implementing some or all of these strategies can help your child develop crucial self-advocacy skills and independence. It will also enable them to communicate their needs better and process the emotional challenges they may face during the school day, because school should be a safe place for kids to learn and grow.

Ask for help and support if your child has emotional support needs that feel too big for you to manage. Mental health professionals can guide you and your child. Don't wait until a problem becomes massive before seeking professional help. For your child's well-being, push past any stigmas you have about seeking professional help.

SELF-ADVOCACY FOR NONSPEAKING CHILDREN

Are you thinking, "Sounds great, but my child is nonspeaking?" Having a nonspeaking child presents different challenges regarding self-advocacy.

Children who are not verbal communicators require trained communication partners. These partners must possess the ability to understand and interpret a child's nonverbal cues, especially when the child cannot or chooses not to use oral language. This understanding is key to being an educated communication partner, enabling adults to decipher signals such as nervous twitching or self-injury. For example, a child who buries their head in their desk and covers their ears might indicate that the environment is too loud for them.

At school, children who can speak have the power to become communication partners to their nonspeaking peers. This empowerment is evident in the following examples:

- Zach was one of two nonspeaking students in a co-taught kindergarten class. The special educator in the class taught the other students to pay attention to Zach's signals when he wanted to play. For instance, she'd narrate things Zach did when other kids were around. "Zach, you picked up your car. Do you want to show it to your friends?" Zach's peers learned that when he picked up an item to show them, it meant he wanted to play.

- Jenni was a second grader who hit her head when the classroom became too loud. At first, Jenni's classmates were shocked and worried when Jenni hit her head. However, Jenni's teacher understood the function of the behavior and explained that "Jenni hits her head when she's trying to tell us it's too loud for her." The other students learned that Jenni needed them to use quieter voices when they saw her bring her hand to her head.

- Jefferson was a third grader with a medical condition that limited his expressive communication and required him to use a wheelchair. His chair was an extension of his body, and he didn't want his classmates to touch it without permission. Jefferson's teacher created a sign that said, "Yes, it's okay to push my wheelchair," and "No, don't touch my wheelchair." She taught the kids how to ask Jefferson if he needed assistance moving around the room. The kids learned to wait for Jefferson to point to yes or no so they'd know whether or not it was okay for them to assist him.

- Maxim was a fifth-grade student who communicated with her peers using an Augmentative and Alternative Communication device, or AAC. To prepare the students for middle school, Maxim's school departmentalized fifth graders to have one teacher for math and science and another for ELA and social studies. Maxim's teachers needed to model how to work collaboratively with Maxim and her peers. Teachers modeled wait time to allow Maxim to respond to other students using her AAC. Learning to provide Maxim with wait time so she could be an active participant rather than a passive one was crucial so that her expressive communication needs didn't limit her from full participation in cooperative classroom activities.

Younger children are naturally curious and eager to help. Preconceived notions do not burden kids, and they are not easily offended, making elementary school the perfect time to teach them how to work and play alongside their nonspeaking peers. This early education fosters inclusive communication and contributes to building a more understanding and supportive future.

Nonspeaking children have different methods of communication. It's helpful for schools to adopt a philosophy of accepting all forms of communication. When school staff respond appropriately to various communication attempts, they strengthen a child's self-advocacy skills. Here are some things you can get the school to pay attention to:

- **Nonverbal Communication:** A child can communicate through body language, eye contact, and physical gestures. Adults should always attempt to acknowledge and understand the child's efforts when they try to convey a message.

- **Assistive Technology Use:** Kids should have access to AAC devices to express their needs and wants. Adults should recognize the child for choosing to communicate using their device to self-advocate.

All communication attempts should be encouraged and supported at school since this validates children. It's also important to understand that sometimes a child will keep trying to communicate using nonverbal cues, while other times, they'll give up.

Always presume competence. This means all children can learn, think, and understand regardless of whether they are verbal or nonspeaking.

SELF-ADVOCACY GOING FORWARD

Building self-advocacy skills is an ongoing process that can take years. It's an ultra-marathon, not a sprint! It's normal for this work to feel hard. You will continue to need to advocate for your child as they progress in school. However, the way your involvement looks should change over time. Remember, you're trying to put yourself out of the job of handling everything for your child so they will develop the self-determination skills they need to thrive. With early and ongoing support, your child will learn to self-advocate for their academic, physical, and social-emotional needs.

> **Tip for Cultivating Joy:** Teaching your child to self-advocate can take a while. Try keeping a Good Things Happen to My Child list to record when you notice your child engaging in self-advocacy. These lists have been popularized online and are usually kept daily. Carve out a regular time to work on your list at least once a week. Five minutes per week can help you build a list that will prove that your child is progressing toward a life of personal agency.

> **Self-Care Tip:** As you teach your child to self-advocate, advocating for your wants and needs is important. One way to do this is by having boundaries and using consistent language to protect your time and space. Beth Ann Mayer interviewed mental health professionals and developed 35 boundary phrases to help you communicate with your children, family, friends, and co-workers. (See Resources.)

Afterword
Take Care of Yourself

At the beginning of this book, I related how my husband and I were wisely advised to care for our marriage while we worked hard at helping our daughter thrive. The warning not to neglect self-care and time as a couple became our guiding light.

What parting words can I offer to persuade *you* to prioritize important relationships and your well-being as you support your child's educational success? Let's start with this.

INTENSIVE PARENTING IS CHALLENGING

Last year, I read about the concept of intensive parenting in *Never Enough: When Achievement Culture Becomes Toxic—and What We Can Do About It* by Jennifer Breheny Wallace. Sociologists define the intensive parenting style as putting the child's needs at the center of family life while the needs of the parents are secondary. Intensive parents sacrifice their own health and well-being when they parent this way. Breheny Wallace interviewed researcher Suniya Luthar, who explained the detriments of intensive parenting in this way:

> But all the ways that we are overstretched—work deadlines, financial anxieties, emotional turmoil, satisfying our child's every need—can deaden our ability to be sensitive, responsive parents. . . . We are more likely to be moody and critical and controlling, and less attuned to our children's emotional cues. Anxiety, depression, and exhaustion impair our perspective and patience, as well as our ability to be consistent; to set healthy boundaries, limits, and schedules; and to find the energy to start fresh the next day when we fall short.

Being a parent is the most demanding job I've ever held, but it's also the most important one. I try not to parent too intensely because I lose myself every time I sacrifice my basic needs for the sake of my children. Luckily, my husband is observant. He encourages me to step away from my computer by 9:00 P.M., giving me at least 90 minutes to unwind with a book in bed before sleep. He takes over bedtime routines when I need an adult time-out, usually consisting of a long shower and blow-drying my hair. He even handles the dishes that accumulate from my stress-baking. Ultimately, he always supports me.

Self-Care Isn't Just Another Task

Many moms often put their own needs last. Whether working inside or outside the home, they juggle a spouse or partner while exhausting themselves to ensure their kids can access various classes, sports, and social activities. Many are part of the sandwich generation who also care for aging parents. I can sense how profoundly tired they are. When I notice a friend in distress, I usually ask, "What are you doing to take care of yourself?" Most of the time, they laugh maniacally or nervously and say, "I don't have time for that." But it's essential, I assure them, because taking care of yourself ultimately benefits the entire family.

Self-care (which many dads need to do better, too!) is not about adding more tasks and appointments to your already busy schedule. Rather, it's about looking for support from others to help you manage it all. Rather than keeping multiple balls in the air, you ask your network of family, friends, or colleagues for help with a couple of them so you have time to do something for yourself to protect your sanity.

IMPORTANT PRINCIPLES FOR SELF-CARE

You've encountered specific self-care tips at the end of each chapter in this book. However, the following are what I consider the overarching principles of my self-care. I hope they'll help you too.

Nurture Adult Friendships

One of the most remarkable ways we can care for ourselves is by nurturing our adult friendships so we don't feel alone on an island with our children. Every adult needs friendship.

As we age, our children, rather than our friends, occupy most of our time. While writing this book, I learned that I'm more productive and a better mom when I take the time to have a meal, or even a coffee, with a friend. The combination of a trusted friend and adult conversation empowers us. Nurturing our friendships provides a support system you may not think you need until you need it.

I've relocated three times since turning 30, and each move has made it harder to forge new friendships. I've found many articles discussing the difficulties of building adult friendships, highlighting that I'm not alone in this struggle.

In "The Easiest Way to Keep Your Friends," Serena Dai suggests setting and sticking to a recurring date to maintain long-term friendships. Arbitrarily trying to schedule dates with two or more friends inevitably leads to logistical hurdles. A recurring calendar event allows you to recreate the time and proximity parameters that were in place when you began your friendship. Plus, a recurring date eliminates the back-and-forth time spent asking when everyone is available.

In her piece, "A Ridiculous, Perfect Way to Make Friends," Mikala Jamison argues that group fitness classes offer an excellent venue for developing adult friendships. These classes focus on a shared passion for exercise, promote regular interaction through consistent attendance, and create opportunities for vulnerability through physical challenges and playful activities. Together, these elements enhance social bonding and ease connections with others. In addition, group fitness classes tackle common obstacles to adult friendships by prompting participants to recognize familiar faces and spark conversations while embracing vulnerability in a nurturing environment. This readiness to connect in a fitness context fosters shared experiences and enhances social confidence in other aspects of life.

I hear you thinking that you don't have the time (or the money or the energy) to do this. I am *not* telling you to join a gym. What I am telling you is that you have to make adult connections. Doing so will allow you to be a better parent since having friendships is an essential part of self-care. You must prioritize your self-care because *your needs matter.*

Be a Selfist

Too often, we deny ourselves the ability to feel refreshed and recharged. Psychologist Carin Rubenstein emphasizes the importance of being a selfist rather than being selfish. A selfist prioritizes personal well-being to support others effectively. This includes taking care of one's physical and mental health, ensuring adequate sleep, enjoying time alone, accepting invitations from friends, and declining engagements that could hinder your well-being. Being a selfist means nurturing your needs *and* those of your family because *your personal needs matter!*

Accept and Offer Help

One of the many things Fred Rogers taught us is "Look for the helpers. You will always find people who are helping." Despite this sage advice (usually applied to disasters and other scary things), many of us have been conditioned to be self-reliant and not to ask for help. A few years after turning 40, I realized we'd gotten it wrong. *There is no shame in asking for help.* Whether you ask your partner to take something off your proverbial plate or reach out to a friend when you feel like one of the 20 plates you're spinning will drop, please get in the habit of asking for help.

We also need to be able to offer help. I may not be able to shovel snow off a neighbor's driveway or help someone unpack boxes when they move, but I am a good cook and love to feed people. You have Covid? I'll drop breakfast off on your porch. You lost a relative? I'll bake something sweet. You had a baby? I'll make you dinner and snacks you can eat when you have the munchies. Dietary restrictions? Tell me what they are and I'll make it work. This is how I help because I know how important it is to be nourished when you feel sick, emotional, or overwhelmed. Plus, I feel happier and less stressed when I can assist someone else.

As Audrey Hepburn said about growing older, "You will discover that you have two hands, one to help yourself and one to help others." You will know which hand you need to use at a given time. I hope you'll come to terms with the fact that this is the time you need the hands of others to support you.

Practice Generosity

In *Infectious Generosity: The Ultimate Idea Worth Spreading,* Chris Anderson, Head of TED, makes the case that everyone can engage in generosity, with or without giving money, by doing little things that can have a ripple effect. We can be generous with our attention, knowledge, skills, or time by sharing one or more things with others. If you're unsure where to begin and don't have time to read the entire book, start with his TED Talk, "It's Time for Infectious Generosity. Here's How." (See Resources.)

This month, challenge yourself to ask for help once and assist someone else once. Start small and be prepared to see the ripple effects.

RESOURCES FOR SELF-CARE

Have you tried out the self-care tips at the end of each chapter? If not, you can try them out at any time. There's a list of them on the book's companion site at *www.guilford.com/shubitz-materials*. And if you're looking for more, check out these resources:

- The Self-Care Wheel created by Olga Phoenix: *https://olgaphoenix.com/self-care-wheel*
- Self-Care Assessment: *www.therapistaid.com/worksheets/self-care-assessment*
- Self-Care Tips: *www.therapistaid.com/worksheets/self-care-tips*

LOOKING AHEAD

As my daughter begins her high school journey, I reflect on that first day of kindergarten—the hand-in-hand journey—and the mix of hope and worry running through me. The path from there to here has been shaped by moments of learning, growth, and a steadfast commitment to supporting her needs. While high school will present new challenges, the foundation we've built through elementary and middle school provides us with a solid base to move onward.

The insights, resources, and strategies shared in this book are tools for you to adapt and use in the days, months, and years ahead. As parents, our role is not to chart their course for our children, but to walk beside them, offering encouragement and support as they forge their own path.

Resources

In the following pages, you'll find a curated list of organizations, resources, and articles that were mentioned in the text or supplement the text. This resource guide is not an exhaustive list in any area, but is merely a starting point.

504 PLANS

- Comparison of the IDEA, Section 504, and the ADA: *www.cadreworks.org/resources/state-resource/id-comparison-idea-section-504-and-ada*
- Frequently Asked Questions About Section 504 and Free Appropriate Public Education (FAPE): *www.ed.gov/laws-and-policy/civil-rights-laws/disability-discrimination/frequently-asked-questions-section-504-fape*
- "What is a 504 Plan?" from the Understood Team: *www.understood.org/articles/what-is-a-504-plan*
- "What Is a 504 Plan? What Teachers and Parents Need to Know" from We Are Teachers: *www.weareteachers.com/what-is-a-504-plan*

ACCESSIBLE MATERIALS

- Bookshare: *www.bookshare.org*
- Learning Ally: *www.learningally.org*
- National Center on Accessible Educational Materials: *https://aem.cast.org*
- The Jewish Braille Institute: *www.jbilibrary.org*
- Texthelp: *www.texthelp.com*

ASSISTIVE TECHNOLOGY

- Myths and Facts Surrounding Assistive Technology Devices and Services, U.S. Department of Education: *https://sites.ed.gov/idea/files/Myths-and-Facts-Surrounding-Assistive-Technology-Devices-01-22-2024.pdf*
- What is assistive technology? *www.understood.org/en/articles/assistive-technology*

BOOK ACCESS

- Apply for National Library Service and Eligibility for Individual Services: *www.loc.gov/nls/how-to-enroll/apply-for-nls-services*
- Hoopla: *www.hoopladigital.com*
- IBBY Collection for Young People with Disabilities: *www.ibby.org/awards-activities/activities/ibby-collection-for-young-people-with-disabilities*
- Learning Ally: *https://learningally.org*
- Libby: *https://libbyapp.com*
- Schneider Family Book Award Lists by Year: *https://library.umw.edu/jyalit/schneider.*
- Sign up for BARD and Access BARD: *www.loc.gov/nls/how-to-enroll/sign-up-for-bard-and-bard-mobile*
- Social Justice Books: Disability: *https://socialjusticebooks.org/booklists/disabilities*

CHARTER SCHOOLS

- National Alliance for Public Charter Schools: *https://publiccharters.org*
- National Charter School Resource Center: *https://charterschoolcenter.ed.gov*
- The Center for Learner Equity, Infographic: Understanding Charter School LEA Status—*www.centerforlearnerequity.org/news/infographic-understanding-charter-school-lea-status/*
- Special Education in Charter Schools: Finding the Right School for Your Child—*www.centerforlearnerequity.org/wp-content/uploads/CLE-Know-Your-Rights-EN.pdf*

CO-TEACHING

- Co-Teaching: A Comprehensive Approach from the New York State Education Department's Office of Special Education: *https://osepartnership.org/pd/A018_Co-Teaching%20A%20ComprehensiveApproach_Module%201.pdf*
- What is Co-Teaching? An Introduction to Co-Teaching and Inclusion from CAST: *https://publishing.cast.org/stories-resources/stories/co-teaching-introduction-inclusion-stein*

DISABILITY EDUCATION

- Hidden Disabilities Sunflower: *https://hdsunflower.com/us*
- Kids Quest: *www.cdc.gov/ncbddd/kids/index.html*

EDUCATION EVALUATIONS

- AAMC: Lower-Cost Evaluation Options: *https://students-residents.aamc.org/applying-medical-school/article/university-clinics*
- How to get a free or low-cost private evaluation: *www.understood.org/en/articles/how-to-get-free-low-cost-evaluation-for-child*
- International Dyslexia Association, Locate a provider for assessment and evaluation: *https://dyslexiaida.org/provider-directories*
- Learning Disabilities Association of America (LDA)
  - State Affiliates Page: *https://ldaamerica.org/support/state-affiliates*
  - Resources: *https://ldaamerica.org/resources/ld-adhd-information-resources*
- National Alliance on Mental Illness (NAMI)
  - You can speak to one of NAMI's volunteer Information and Resource Referral Specialists. Call the NAMI HelpLine at 800-950-NAMI (6264).
- School *Services* for Children with Special Needs: Know Your Rights
  - *www.aacap.org/AACAP/Families_and_Youth/Facts_for_Families/FFF-Guide/Services-In-School-For-Children-With-Special-Needs-What-Parents-Need-To-Know-083.aspx*
- Who Can Diagnose LD and/or ADHD: *www.readingrockets.org/topics/assessment-and-evaluation/articles/who-can-diagnose-ld-andor-adhd*

FAMILY TIME ACTIVITY FINDER

- AllEvents: *https://allevents.in*
- Clipp: *www.clipp.com*
- Groupon: *www.groupon.com*
- Mommy Poppins—"What should I do today?": *https://mommypoppins.com/anywhere-family/what-should-i-do-today*
- Tripadvisor: *www.tripadvisor.com*

FAPE

- IEP vs. 504 Plan: *www.weareteachers.com/what-is-a-504-plan*
- IDEA: Explanations of the 13 specific disabilities one must have to get an IEP: *https://sites.ed.gov/idea/regs/b/a/300.8*

HOMEWORK

- Alfie Kohn's Articles, Arranged by Periodical: *www.alfiekohn.org/articles*
- Two Writing Teachers—Homework Mini Series: *https://twowritingteachers.org/2017/11/20/recap-hmwkmini*

IDEA

- Code of Federal Regulations, 300.8 Child with a Disability: *www.ecfr.gov/current/title-34/subtitle-B/chapter-III/part-300/subpart-A/subject-group-ECFR0ec59c730ac278e/section-300.8*
- Questions and Answers on Serving Children with Disabilities Placed by Their Parents in Private Schools: *https://sites.ed.gov/idea/files/QA_on_Private_Schools_02-28-2022.pdf.*
- Sec. 300.34 Related services: *https://sites.ed.gov/idea/regs/b/a/300.34*
- Sec. 300.518 Child's status during proceedings: *https://sites.ed.gov/idea/regs/b/e/300.518*

JOURNALING

- 10 Journaling Tips to Help You Heal, Grow and Thrive: *https://tinybuddha*
  .com/blog/10-journaling-tips-to-help-you-heal-grow-and-thrive
- Journaling for Emotional Wellness: *www.urmc.rochester.edu/encyclopedia/*
  content.aspx?ContentID=4552&ContentTypeID=1
- The Beginner's Guide to Benefits of Journaling and How to Start Writing:
  www.oprahdaily.com/life/a35231175/how-to-start-a-journal

JOY

- Greater Good Resources for Summer Fun: *https://greatergood.berkeley.edu/*
  article/item/greater_good_resources_for_summer_fun
- One Question for a More Joyful Day: *https://aestheticsofjoy.com/one-question*
  -for-a-more-joyful-day
- The Poem Farm: *https://poemfarm.amylv.com*
- Three Good Things: *https://ggia.berkeley.edu/practice/three-good-things*
- Watch Louie Schwartzberg's TED Talk: *www.ted.com/talks/louie_schwartz-*
  berg_nature_beauty_gratitude

LEAST RESTRICTIVE ENVIRONMENT

- Least Restrictive Environment (LRE) Under the Individuals with
  Disabilities Education Act (IDEA): *www.advocacydenver.org/resources/for*
  *-children/*least-restrictive-environment
- Starter Set of Resources on LRE from Center for Parent Information and
  Resources: *www.parentcenterhub.org/lre-resources*

LEGAL

Advocacy and Attorneys

- Council of Parent Attorneys and Advocates (COPAA) Member Directory:
  www.copaa.org/page/Direct

- National Disability Rights Network: *www.ndrn.org*
- The Advocacy Institute: *www.advocacyinstitute.org*
- The Center for Appropriate Dispute Resolution in Special Education: *www.cadreworks.org*

Due Process Hearing

- IDEA Special Education Due Process Complaints Parent Guide: *www.cadreworks.org/resources/cadre-materials/idea-dispute-resolution-parent-guides/due-process-complaints*
- Impartial due process hearing: *https://sites.ed.gov/idea/regs/b/e/300.511*
- Quick Guide to Special Education Dispute Resolution Processes for Parents of Children and Youth (Ages 3–21): *www.cadreworks.org/resources/cadre-materials/quick-guide-special-education-dispute-resolution-processes-parents*
- The Due Process Complaint in Part B of IDEA: *www.parentcenterhub.org/dueprocess*
- The Due Process Hearing, in Detail: *www.parentcenterhub.org/details-due-process/#:~:text=During%20a%20due%20process%20hearing,the%20issues%20in%20the%20hearing*
- What to expect at a due process hearing: *www.understood.org/articles/what-to-expect-at-a-due-process-hearing*

Mediation

- IDEA Special Education Mediation Parent Guide: *www.cadreworks.org/resources/cadre-materials/idea-dispute-resolution-parent-guides/mediation*
- Mediation under Part B of IDEA: *www.parentcenterhub.org/mediation*

OCR Complaints

- How the Office for Civil Rights Handles Complaints: *www2.ed.gov/about/offices/list/ocr/complaints-how.html*
- How to File a Discrimination Complaint with the Office for Civil Rights: *www2.ed.gov/about/offices/list/ocr/docs/howto.pdf*
- OCR Discrimination Complaint Form: *www.ed.gov/laws-and-policy/civil-rights-laws/file-complaint/ocr-discrimination-complaint-form*

Sample P&A Goals and Objectives

• Minnesota Disability Law Center's Statement of Goals and Priorities: *https://mylegalaid.org/wp-content/uploads/2024/02/Final-MDLC-2024-Priorities.pdf*

State Complaints

• Filing a State Complaint in Part B of IDEA: *www.parentcenterhub.org/statecomplaint*

  ○ IDEA Special Education Written State Complaints Parent Guide: *www.cadreworks.org/resources/cadre-materials/idea-dispute-resolution-parent-guides/written-state-complaints*

  ○ IDEA State Complaint Resource Center: *www.advocacyinstitute.org/iscrc/index.shtml*

  ○ What to include in a state complaint for IEP dispute resolution: *www.understood.org/articles/what-to-include-in-a-state-complaint*

MENTAL HEALTH

• Anxiety Aid Tools: *https://anxietyaidtools.com*
• National Alliance on Mental Illness: *www.nami.org*
• The Jed Foundation: *https://jedfoundation.org/mental-health-resource-center*

MINDFULNESS

• Mindfulness for Kids: *www.mindful.org/mindfulness-for-kids*
• Positive Psychology: *https://positivepsychology.com/mindfulness-for-children-kids-activities*
• Susan Kaiser Greenland's Mindfulness Games: *https://susankaisergreenland.com/videos-for-educators#mindfulgames*

NATIONAL ORGANIZATIONS

• Center for Parent Information and Resources: *www.parentcenterhub.org/find-your-center*
• Family-to-Family Health Information Centers: *https://familyvoices.org*

- National Federation of Families: *www.ffcmh.org/our-affiliates*
- Parent To Parent USA: *www.p2pusa.org/parents*
- The Arc: *https://thearc.org*

NEURODIVERSITY TERMINOLOGY GLOSSARIES

- Glossary Reframing Autism: *https://reframingautism.org.au/service/glossary -terms*
- Neuroqueer's key neurodiversity-related terminology, their meanings, proper usage, and misusage: *https://neuroqueer.com/neurodiversity-terms-and -definitions*
- Weirdly Successful's Neurodivergent Glossary—Big Book of Terms: *https:// weirdlysuccessful.org/glossary*

PLAY

- National Institute for Play: How We Play: *www.nifplay.org/what-is-play/ types-of-play*
- PDF Tips from Challenge Success: *https://challengesuccess.org/resources/pdf -tips*
- Why Play?: *https://learningthroughplay.com/why-play*

SELF-CARE

- 35 Phrases To Set Boundaries Firmly and Fairly, According to Mental Health Pros: *https://parade.com/living/boundary-phrases*
- Breathing exercises to reduce stress: *www.headspace.com/meditation/breathing -exercises*
- How Box Breathing Can Help You Destress: *https://health.clevelandclinic.org /box-breathing-benefits*
- How Holding Yourself Can Reduce Stress: *https://greatergood.berkeley.edu/ podcasts/item/how_holding_yourself_can_reduce_stress_calvin_cato*

- How To Show Up For Yourself: *https://greatergood.berkeley.edu/podcasts/item/self_compassionate_touch_brittany_luse*
- It's Time for Infectious Generosity. Here's How: *www.youtube.com/watch?app=desktop&v=I1ouTj1BQec*
- Self-Care Assessment: *www.therapistaid.com/worksheets/self-care-assessment*
- Self-Care Tips: *www.therapistaid.com/worksheets/self-care-tips*
- The Self-Care Wheel created by Olga Phoenix: *https://olgaphoenix.com/self-care-wheel*

SMART GOALS

- How to tell if your child's IEP goals are SMART: *www.understood.org/en/articles/how-to-tell-if-your-childs-iep-goals-are-smart*
- SMART IEPs: *www.wrightslaw.com/bks/feta2/ch12.ieps.pdf*
- What are SMART Goals in Education? *www.twinkl.com/teaching-wiki/smart-goals-in-education*

SOCIAL AND EMOTIONAL LEARNING

- Collaborative for Academic, Social, and Emotional Learning (CASEL): *https://casel.org*
- Committee for Children: *www.cfchildren.org*
- Conversation Cards about Emotions: *www.mightier.com/resources/conversation-cards-about-emotions-by-mightier*
- From a Nation at Risk to a Nation at Home: Recommendations from the National Commission on Social, Emotional, & Academic Development: *www.aspeninstitute.org/wp-content/uploads/2023/02/Nation-at-Hope.pdf*
- How Can We Help Kids With Self-Regulation? *https://childmind.org/article/can-help-kids-self-regulation*
- Research & the Zones of Regulation: *https://zonesofregulation.com/research*
- Responsive Classroom: *www.responsiveclassroom.org*
- RULER (Yale Center for Emotional Intelligence): *https://rulerapproach.org*

SPECIAL EDUCATION TEACHER SHORTAGE

- High Standards & Innovative Solutions: How Some States are Addressing the Special Educator Shortage Crisis: *https://sites.ed.gov/osers/2023/05/high-standards-innovative-solutions-how-some-states-are-addressing-the-special-educator-shortage-crisis*
- Retention Is the Missing Ingredient in Special Education Staffing: *www.edweek.org/leadership/retention-is-the-missing-ingredient-in-special-education-staffing/2024/05*
- What Schools Can Do about the Special Ed Teacher Shortage: *www.bu.edu/wheelock/news/articles/2024/what-schools-can-do-about-the-special-education-teacher-shortage*
- What Will Teacher Shortages Look Like in 2024 and Beyond? A Researcher Weighs In: *www.edweek.org/leadership/what-will-teacher-shortages-look-like-in-2024-and-beyond-a-researcher-weighs-in/2023/12*
- What's driving a special education teacher shortage and how schools are responding: *www.pbs.org/newshour/show/whats-driving-a-special-education-teacher-shortage-and-how-schools-are-responding*
- Why children with disabilities are missing school and losing skills: *www.npr.org/2024/05/15/1247795768/children-disabilities-special-education-teacher-shortage*

SUMMER CAMPS

- American Camp Association: Find a Camp: *https://find.acacamps.org*
- Summer 365: Children 7-12: *www.summer365.com/camps-and-experiences/children-7-12/*
- The Camp Experts: *www.campexperts.com/special-needs-camp*

SUPPLEMENTARY AIDS AND SERVICES

- The Short Story on Supplementary Aids and Services: *www.parentcenterhub.org/iep-supplementary/#short*

TEACHER SHORTAGE

- High Standards & Innovative Solutions: How Some States are Addressing the Special Educator Shortage Crisis: *https://sites.ed.gov/osers/2023/05/high -standards-innovative-solutions-how-some-states-are-addressing-the-special-educator -shortage-crisis*

- Retention Is the Missing Ingredient in Special Education Staffing: *www .edweek.org/leadership/retention-is-the-missing-ingredient-in-special-education-staff- ing/2024/05*

- What Schools Can Do about the Special Ed Teacher Shortage: *www.bu.edu /wheelock/news/articles/2024/what-schools-can-do-about-the-special-education -teacher-shortage*

- What Will Teacher Shortages Look Like in 2024 and Beyond? A Researcher Weighs In: *www.edweek.org/leadership/what-will-teacher-shortages -look-like-in-2024-and-beyond-a-researcher-weighs-in/2023/12*

- What's driving a special education teacher shortage and how schools are responding: *www.pbs.org/newshour/show/whats-driving-a-special-education -teacher-shortage-and-how-schools-are-responding*

- Why children with disabilities are missing school and losing skills: *www.npr .org/2024/05/15/1247795768/children-disabilities-special-education-teacher -shortage*

UNIVERSAL DESIGN

- Center for Applied Special Technology (CAST): *www.cast.org*
- Parent Advocacy Brief from the National Center for Learning Disabilities: A Parent's Guide to UDL: *www.advocacyinstitute.org/resources/ ParentUDLGuide.pdf*

References

Introduction

Yu, T. 2024. *The Anti-Ableist Manifesto: Smashing Stereotypes, Forging Change, and Building a Disability-Inclusive World*. New York: Hachette Go.

Chapter 1

Bergland, C. 2019. Longer Exhalations Are an Easy Way to Hack Your Vagus Nerve. *Psychology Today*. First published online May 9, 2019. *www.psychologytoday.com/us/blog/the-athletes-way/201905/longer-exhalations-are-easy-way-hack-your-vagus-nerve*.

Cleveland Clinic. 2021. How Box Breathing Can Help You Destress. First published online August 17, 2021. *https://health.clevelandclinic.org/box-breathing-benefits*.

Headspace. n.d. Breathing Exercises to Reduce Stress. *www.headspace.com/meditation/breathing-exercises*.

Ladau, E. 2021. *Demystifying Disability: What to Know, What to Say, and How to Be an Ally*. New York: Ten Speed Press.

Meehan, M. 2020. *Every Child Can Write: Entry Points, Bridges and Pathways for Striving Writers*. Thousand Oaks, CA: Corwin Literacy.

Shew, A. 2023. *Against Technoableism: Rethinking Who Needs Improvement*. New York: W.W. Norton.

The World Bank. 2023. Disability Inclusion. Last updated April 3, 2023. *www.worldbank.org/en/topic/disability*.

Chapter 2

Individuals with Disabilities Education Act. 2018. Sec. 300.8 Child with a Disability. Last updated May 25, 2018. *https://sites.ed.gov/idea/regs/b/a/300.8*.

Chapter 3

Hehir, T. 2017. Academic Modifications: What You Need to Know. Understood. *https://youtu.be/tuKdIxmd6QE?si=9Uytbcc2B-lKBGm3*.

Individuals with Disabilities Education Act. 2017. Sec. 300.34 Related Services. Last updated May 2, 2017. *https://sites.ed.gov/idea/regs/b/a/300.34.*

Chapter 4

Friend, M. 2020. *Interactions: Collaboration Skills for School Professionals.* 9th ed. Hoboken, NJ: Pearson.

Haas, S. B. (2019). Working with Your Hands Does Wonders for Your Brain. Psychology Today. June 21. *www.psychologytoday.com/us/blog/prescriptions-life/201906/working-your-hands-does-wonders-your-brain.*

Jung, L., D. Frey, J. Fisher, and J. Kroener. 2019. *Your Students, My Students, Our Students: Rethinking Equitable and Inclusive Classrooms.* Arlington, VA: ASCD.

National Center for Education Statistics. 2023. Students With Disabilities. Condition of Education. U.S. Department of Education, Institute of Education Sciences. Accessed February 17, 2023. *https://nces.ed.gov/programs/coe/indicator/cgg.*

Ross, L. J. 2019. Speaking Up without Tearing Down. Teaching Tolerance Magazine 61 (Spring): 19–22.

Yu, T. 2024. The Anti-Ableist Manifesto: Smashing Stereotypes, Forging Change, and Building a Disability-Inclusive World. New York: Hachette Go.

Individuals with Disabilities Education Act. 2017. Sec. 300.114 LRE Requirements. Last updated May 3, 2017. *https://sites.ed.gov/idea/regs/b/b/300.114.*

Chapter 5

Brous, S. 2024. *The Amen Effect: Ancient Wisdom to Mend Our Broken Hearts and the World.* New York: Penguin Random House.

Individuals with Disabilities Education Act. 2017. Sec. 300.39 (b) (3). Last updated May 2, 2017. *https://sites.ed.gov/idea/regs/b/a/300.39/b/3.*

Pryal, K. R. G. 2023. Accommodations and Accessibility: What's the Difference? Psychology Today. November 6. *www.psychologytoday.com/us/blog/living-neurodivergence/202310/accommodations-and-accessibility-whats-the-difference.*

Chapter 7

Cleveland Clinic. 2020. 3 Reasons Adult Coloring Can Actually Relax Your Brain. May 26. *https://health.clevelandclinic.org/3-reasons-adult-coloring-can-actually-relax-brain.*

Chapter 8

Anbar, R. D. 2024. 3 Activities to Beneficially Release Dopamine. *Psychology Today. www.psychologytoday.com/us/blog/understanding-hypnosis/202402/3-activities-to-beneficially-release-dopamine.*

Brooks, A. C. 2024. Busyness, Boredom, and the Perils of Always Being in Motion. *The Atlantic,* April 18. *www.theatlantic.com/ideas/archive/2024/04/busyness-boredom-happiness-worklife/678085.*

Cherry, K. 2024. 10 Surprising Psychological Benefits of Music. Verywell Mind. *www. verywellmind.com/surprising-psychological-benefits-of-music-4126866.*

Duke, N. 2022. What Wordle Reminds Us About Effective Phonics and Spelling Instruction. ASCD Blog. *https://ascd.org/blogs/what-wordle-reminds-us-about-effective-phonics-and -spelling-instruction.*

Garey, J. 2024. The Power of Mindfulness. Child Mind Institute. *https://childmind.org/article /the-power-of-mindfulness.*

Kohn, A. 2006. *The Homework Myth: Why Our Kids Get Too Much of a Bad Thing.* Philadelphia: Da Capo Press.

Kohn. A. 2012. The Case Against Homework. *Family Circle. www.alfiekohn.org/article/case -against-homework.*

Lee, I. F. 2018. *Joyful: The Surprising Power of Ordinary Things to Create Extraordinary Happiness.* New York: Little, Brown Spark.

LEGO Foundation and Tænketanken Mandag Morgen. (2021). The Good Life – According to Children. *https://cde-lego-cms-prod.azureedge.net/media/r4nd0vq4/tmm-det-gode-b%C3 %B8meliv_en_gb_lowres.pdf.*

Miller, D. 2017. Access to Books: A Game Changer for Kids. Keynote at Teachers College, February 9, 2017.

Pietrangelo, A. 2019. How Does Dopamine Affect the Body? *Healthline. www.healthline.com /health/dopamine-effects.*

UMass Memorial Health Center for Mindfulness. n.d. Mindfulness Programs FAQ's. *www. ummhealth.org/umass-memorial-medical-center/services-treatments/center-for-mindfulness/faqs.*

United Nations Human Rights: Office of the High Commissioner. n.d. Convention on the Rights of the Child | OHCHR. *www.ohchr.org/en/instruments-mechanisms/instruments/ convention-rights-child.*

Wood, S. 2022. Should Kids Get Homework? *U.S. News and World Report. www.usnews.com /education/k12/articles/should-kids-get-homework.*

Chapter 9

Bishop R. S. 1990. Mirrors, Windows, and Sliding Glass Doors. *Perspectives 6* (3): ix–xi.

Grabmeier, J. 2019. *The Importance of Reading to Kids Daily.* The Ohio State University College of Education and Human Ecology, April 9. *https://ehe.osu.edu/news/listing/ importance-reading-kids-daily-0.*

Jackson–Retondo, M. 2023. Choosing Children's Books That Include and Affirm Disability Experiences. KQED, August 7. *www.kqed.org/mindshift/62049/choosing-childrens-books -that-include-and-affirm-disability-experiences.*

Chapter 10

CASEL. 2021. SEL 101: What Are the Core Competencies and Key Settings? YouTube Video, June 23. *https://youtu.be/ouXhi_CfBVg?si=g4vZXnvexsSzIREi.*

Mayer, B. A. 2023. 35 Phrases To Set Boundaries Firmly and Fairly, According to Mental Health *Pros. Parade,* May 12. *https://parade.com/living/boundary-phrases*

Test, D. W., C. H. Fowler, W. M. Wood, D. M. Brewer, and S. Eddy. 2005. A Conceptual Framework of Self-Advocacy for Students with Disabilities. Remedial and Special Education 26 (1): 43–54.

University of New Hampshire. n.d. What Is Self-Advocacy? Diversity, Equity, Access and Inclusion. *www.unh.edu/diversity-inclusion/student-accessibility/students/self-advocacy-guide/what-self-advocacy*.

Afterword

Anderson, C. 2024. *Infectious Generosity: The Ultimate Idea Worth Spreading*. New York: Crown.

Breheny Wallace, J. 2023. *Never Enough: When Achievement Culture Becomes Toxic–and What We Can Do About It*. New York: Portfolio / Penguin.

Dai, S. 2025. The Easiest Way to Keep Your Friends. *The Atlantic*, January 12. *www.theatlantic.com/family/archive/2025/01/friendship-schedule-recurring-calendar-date/681292*.

Jamison, M. 2024. A Ridiculous, Perfect Way to Make Friends. *The Atlantic*, November 20. *www.theatlantic.com/health/archive/2024/11/group-fitness-exercise-friendship/680713*.

Index

Note: 't' and 'f' denotes tables and figures respectively

About the Author

Stacey Shubitz, MSEd, MA, is a certified literacy specialist and former fourth- and fifth-grade teacher in the New York City Public Schools and a public charter school in Rhode Island. Since 2009, she has been a literacy consultant, supporting teachers with writing instruction. Stacey has published several books, including *Welcome to Writing Workshop: Engaging Today's Students* and *Craft Moves: Lesson Sets for Teaching Writing.* She holds an MA in Literacy Education from Teachers College at Columbia University and an MSEd in Childhood Education from Hunter College. Stacey co-founded the Two Writing Teachers blog in 2007 and co-hosts the Two Writing Teachers Podcast.